RxEAD THE PRESCRIPTION LABEL

And Other Tips to Prevent Deadly and Costly Medication Errors

Mary Sue McAslan, Pharm.D.

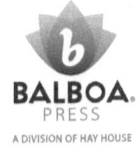

BALBOA.
PRESS

A DIVISION OF HAY HOUSE

ISBN: 978-1-4525-4722-0 (sc)
ISBN: 978-1-4525-4723-7 (e)

Balboa Press books may be ordered through booksellers or by contacting:

Balboa Press
A Division of Hay House
1663 Liberty Drive
Bloomington, IN 47403
www.balboapress.com
1-(877) 407-4847

Because of the dynamic nature of the Internet, any web addresses or links contained in this book may have changed since publication and may no longer be valid. The views expressed in this work are solely those of the author and do not necessarily reflect the views of the publisher, and the publisher hereby disclaims any responsibility for them.

The author of this book does not dispense medical advice or prescribe the use of any technique as a form of treatment for physical, emotional, or medical problems without the advice of a physician, either directly or indirectly. The intent of the author is only to offer information of a general nature to help you in your quest for medical wellbeing. In the event you use any of the information in this book for yourself, which is your constitutional right, the author and the publisher assume no responsibility for your actions.

Any people depicted in stock imagery provided by Thinkstock are models, and such images are being used for illustrative purposes only.
Certain stock imagery © Thinkstock.

Printed in the United States of America

Balboa Press rev. date:3/21/2012

To Mom: pharmacist, advocate, and caregiver

Contents

Part 4. The Successful Hospital Stay: Preventing Medication Errors in the Hospital _____ 105

Introduction

Imagine that you are reading the newspaper on Monday morning and the headline reads, "Fully Loaded Jumbo Jet Crashes with 200 Passengers on Board. All Are Dead." Then imagine that you are reading the newspaper on Wednesday morning and the headline again reads, "Fully Loaded Jumbo Jet Crashes with 200 Passengers on Board. All Are Dead." Imagine that this headline repeats every other day of every week of every year!

How long do you think it would take the airline industry to respond to catastrophes of this magnitude?

How long before you stopped flying?

How long before Congress would hold hearings on airline safety?

How long would you put up with this?

In 1999, the Institute of Medicine (IOM) published a report called "To Err Is Human: Building a Safer Health System."[1] In this report, the IOM identified a very large and serious problem that doctors, pharmacists, nurses, and other health-care providers were making mistakes. The IOM report estimated that medical mistakes were killing nearly ninety-eight thousand people every year, or the equivalent of three fully loaded jumbo jets crashing every other day.

The 1999 IOM report caused a big stir in the media. All the major news networks covered it extensively: CNN, the *LA Times*, and others. The report called for a 50 percent reduction in medical errors in the next five years. As a result, a federal task force examined medical errors and confirmed the IOM's findings. The report also recommended that there should be a national focus to increase patient safety, develop a mandatory national reporting system for medical errors, raise performance standards for safety, and implement safety systems—especially for the delivery of medications.

However, once the initial outrage from the IOM report faded, the media and the government moved on to other issues. In 2004, five years after the initial report, no major changes in medical error reporting had occurred and other changes in our health-care system remained "frustratingly slow."[2]

In May 2009, ten years after the release of the initial IOM report, the Consumer's Union (CU) released a follow-up report. This report was called, "To Err Is Human—To Delay Is Deadly. Ten Years Later, a Million Lives Lost, Billions of Dollars Wasted." [3] What the Consumer's Union found was that *preventable* medical harm still accounted for more than one hundred thousand deaths each year or a million lives over the past decade. Additionally, the CU noted that by all accounts this statistic was conservative. On creating a health-care system that was free of preventable medical harm, the Consumer's Union gave the country a failing grade.

In addition to the cost in human life, medical mistakes cost billions in health-care dollars. The 1999 IOM report estimated that medical errors cost the United States $17–$29 billion every year.[4] Statistics related to medical mistakes are hard to measure and evaluate; however, the consensus appears to be that we are no safer today than we were ten years ago.

Medication Errors: What They Are and Why They Happen

Estimates show that over 1.5 million medication errors happen every year in the United States and figures suggest that on average, every hospital patient has one medication administration error every day.[5] Most of these errors are not fatal; they are what we call "near misses." Although near misses are mistakes that do not cause permanent injury or death, they may lead to needless and preventable hospitalizations or disability. Unfortunately, there are medication errors that cause fatalities. The Institute of Medicine concluded that seven thousand people die needlessly each year due to medication errors.[6]

Medication errors include the following:

- ➢ getting the wrong drug
- ➢ getting the wrong dose
- ➢ getting the wrong directions
- ➢ getting two drugs that interact with each other
- ➢ getting a drug you are allergic to
- ➢ getting a drug meant for someone else

As a pharmacist with over thirty years experience specializing in medication errors, I have seen countless numbers of needless, preventable mistakes. In my career, I have also seen many quality improvement initiatives come and go, numerous safe practice standards put into place and fail, and state-of-the-art computer systems that actually *cause* medication errors rather than prevent them. I can safely say that we have had a definite problem in our health-care system for over three decades, and the problem is not going away.

Preventing Medication Errors: The New and Critical Role of the Patient

The 1999 IOM report highlighted the fragmented nature of health-care delivery in our country and the critical role patients play in providing their doctors with important information related to their medication therapy.

The IOM report stated, "Patients themselves could provide a major safety check in most hospitals, clinics and practices. They should know which medications they are taking, their appearance, and their side effects, and they should notify their doctors of medication discrepancies and the occurrence of side effects."[7]

This represents a new role for the patient and caregiver. It will require a change in the way we have always done things. In the past, we have subscribed to the notion that our doctors, pharmacists, and nurses knew everything about and coordinated our entire health care. The results from the IOM report clearly showed that this is not the case, and medication errors are continuing to occur at an alarming rate. As a patient taking an active role in your own care, you must be willing to challenge the "way we have always done things" and start to use the solutions in this book to reduce medication errors and harm.

How to Use This Book

This book contains sixty different safety tips to help you prevent medication errors at the doctor's office, the pharmacy, the hospital, and at home. It is not meant to be read all at once. You should refer to it during each step of your medical care.

Each safety tip is written in the same format. This includes a brief description of the safety issue followed by a lifelike story and "Rxpert Advice" where I provide simple solutions for preventing errors. Lastly, you will see the "Bottom Line," which provides you with the most important facts in a quick and easy format. Certain safety tips contain links to my website (www.drmarysue.com) where you will find free downloads and other important safety information.

Each safety tip in this book includes a story. The stories are a compilation of adaptations based upon over thirty years of my personal experience. They are provided to illustrate the principles presented in the safety tip, help you understand and remember complicated information, and then encourage you to take action to prevent an error from happening to you or someone you care for. Any similarities to actual events are strictly coincidental. In some cases, I use medications by their brand names because I believe that this is the most familiar and helpful way for you to understand the information. I have no connection to any drug companies, especially those whose products are listed in this book.

If you find yourself questioning my advice—and it will happen—keep reading; there are hundreds of points and observations in this book. You do not have to accept all of them. Additionally, discuss the information in this book with your doctor and pharmacist; they can provide additional clarification and feedback.

Many of the tips in this book are my subjective opinion, but they are based on years of research and professional experience. Some tips may cause you concern or some level of discomfort. Do not discount the tips that make you uncomfortable. It just may be that the point applies to you and hits too close to home.

This book is not for those people who are completely satisfied with the quality and safety of their health care. I wrote this book for people who are serious about taking meaningful steps to prevent medication errors from happening to themselves or someone they love or care for.

There are numerous books written by experts telling you what you need to do to prevent medical mistakes. I did not want to write another book about alarming mistakes and provide you with nothing more than generalities and platitudes that have no real application to your life. Done right, this book should energize you and give you functional, doable things to make your health care safer. This book is based upon doing things differently, most notably, taking an active role in understanding your medication therapy and other treatment plans.

Refer to your doctor and other health-care providers (specialists, dentists, pharmacists, and nurses) for specific medical advice. They are the experts in your medical care. This book should in no way be used as a substitute for advice from your medical professional or legal counsel.

In referring to your doctor, I have used the term "he" for simplicity. The term includes all doctors male and female. Medication is also referred to as med, medicine, drug, and pill interchangeably.

If you are truly serious about preventing medication errors, then let's get to work.

Part 1

Preventing Medication Errors: It's Up to You

Medication errors happen every day in our hospitals, doctor's offices, pharmacies, and homes. The number of errors is overwhelming. However, what most people don't know is that most of these errors can be prevented. Serious harm can be avoided if the patient or the caregiver speaks up, asks questions, and gets the necessary answers before proceeding with any medication or treatment.

I often tell a person that if you think that there's been a mistake, trust your gut—speak up and ask questions. However, many people are intimidated by their doctor or don't even know what questions to ask. In this section, I will give you four questions to ask every time your doctor, nurse, or pharmacist gives you a new medication.

Preventing medication errors also includes keeping complete and up-to-date health records. I will show you exactly how to keep a medication list and organize your other records using the Personal Health System.

The first five safety tips apply to every aspect and circumstance of your health care. Read these tips first and refer back to them as a refresher before your doctor appointments or hospitalizations.

Knowing that it is up to you to trust your gut, speak up, and ask questions is critical to preventing serious medication errors from happening to you or someone you care for.

You, the patient, are the last line of defense against medication errors.

Safety Tip #1
Trust Your Gut: If It Doesn't Seem Right, It Probably Isn't

The most important thing that you can do to prevent a serious medication error is to learn to trust your gut feeling. If something does not seem right to you, it probably isn't and there may have been a mistake.

Many victims of medication errors say that they knew something just didn't seem right, but they took the pills anyway. Most admit that they could have prevented a mistake from happening if they would have just asked questions and gotten the problem cleared up before taking the drug. This tip applies to all areas of your health care, including the hospital, the pharmacy, the doctor's office, and at home.

"It Just Didn't Seem Right"

Bob had a heart condition, and his doctor prescribed a medication to thin his blood. Bob had taken this medicine for years and led a completely normal life. He went to the lab to get his blood tested once a month. He never worried; his blood always tested normal.

This month, Bob had his blood tested and as usual went about his day, running some errands while he waited for the nurse to call him with the results. Carolyn, his wife, answered the phone when the nurse called, and to the best of her ability she wrote down the instructions the nurse gave her.

"Bob's blood test is fine," the nurse said. "He should continue to take his blood thinner as usual. He should take a 4 mg pill on Monday, Wednesday, and Friday, and a 5 mg pill on Sunday, Tuesday, Thursday, and Saturday."

What Carolyn wrote down was, "Take 4 pills on Monday, Wednesday, and Friday and take 5 pills on Sunday, Tuesday, Thursday, and Saturday."

When Bob came home, he read the instructions Carolyn had written down. Bob thought *That just doesn't seem right*, because he had never taken that many blood thinner pills before, yet he did exactly as his wife told him.

A few days later, Bob noticed several new bruises on his arms. He also noticed that his gums bled when he brushed his teeth. Bob knew that these were the signs of taking too much blood thinner, and he was scared. He thought it would be a good idea to call his doctor. Bob was right.

The doctor told Bob to come into his office right away. He needed to do a blood test to measure how thin Bob's blood was. When Bob told his doctor how he had been taking his blood thinner—five pills one day, then four pills the next day—the doctor became very concerned about an overdose and admitted him to the hospital, where he stayed until his blood returned to normal.

Bob had learned his lesson the hard way. From now on, if something about his blood thinner did not seem right, he was going to call his doctor or nurse to clear things up before he took the pill.

R_xpert Advice

➢ If anything about your prescription medicine does not seem right to you, such as

➢ the name on the bottle;

➢ the color, shape, or size of the pill;

➢ the number of pills;

➢ the directions; or

➢ the reason you are taking it,

then it probably isn't.

Stop, ask questions, and get the answers you need before taking the medication.

> ➤ The Joint Commission on the Accreditation of Healthcare Organizations (JCAHO) Speak Up Program offers consumers easy-to-read information to prevent medical mistakes.[8] Check out their website at www.jointcommission.org.

> ➤ In safety tip #3, I will provide you with four questions to ask your doctor, nurse, or pharmacist. These will help you to get the information you need to take your medications safely.

Bottom Line

Learn to trust your gut. If something doesn't seem right about your medications, or any other area of your health care, *stop*, speak up, ask questions, and get the answers you need. You could be preventing a serious medication error.

Safety Tip #2
Assumptions Kill: Never Assume Anything

When it comes to your health care, never assume anything. This is especially true if you see several doctors and other health-care providers (nurses, therapists, etc.). There may be a lack of communication between your doctor and your other providers.

Lack of communication can lead to serious errors, including the following:

- getting two or more drugs that do exactly the same thing
- getting two drugs that interact with each other
- getting a drug that you are allergic to

Never assume anything, including that there has been adequate communication between all of the health-care providers that take care of you. It is up to you to ask questions and understand the information that your doctors give you. It is also up to you to notify your doctor of any new medications that another doctor prescribed for you. Again, never assume anything. This could save your life.

"I'm Deathly Allergic to Penicillin"

Late one evening my friend Joanne came into the pharmacy where I was working. Joanne's dentist had called in a prescription from his home. The prescription was for penicillin, which she was to take before her dental appointment the next morning. While preparing the prescription, I noticed that I did not have a record of Joanne's medication allergies in the pharmacy computer. I said, "Joanne, are you allergic to any medications?" "Oh yes!" she said. "I'm deathly allergic to penicillin. The last time I took it, I nearly stopped breathing."

I told her that the prescription her dentist had called in was for penicillin and that I would need to contact him to have it changed. I called the dentist and notified him of the allergy. The dentist had no record of the allergy since he was calling from home. He was extremely grateful that I had asked about Joanne's allergies. We narrowly averted what could have been a life-threatening mistake.

Joanne had assumed that her dentist knew she was allergic to penicillin. Joanne also assumed that I had a record of her allergies in the pharmacy computer. Both of these assumptions were wrong and could have proved deadly. Joanne swore that she would take extra precautions from now on to remind her doctors, dentist, pharmacist, and other health-care providers of her penicillin allergy.

R$_x$pert Advice

> Do not assume that each of your doctors and other health-care providers has a complete and updated list of your medical issues, medications, or medication allergies. This is especially true if you have new medications prescribed by another doctor or allergies that have recently surfaced.

> In safety tip # 4, I show you how to prepare a medication list that you can take to each doctor's appointment. This is a list of all of your medications, including prescriptions and over-the-counter drugs. It also has a place to write your medication allergies. It is up to you to update this list and review it with your doctor at each visit.

Bottom Line

Never assume that all of your health-care providers have your complete and accurate medical information. It is up to you to make sure they have the information they need.

Safety Tip #3
There's No Such Thing as
a Stupid Question

Have you ever left the doctor's office with a new prescription in hand and no clue in your mind about the name of the drug, why you were taking it, how you were supposed to take it, or the side effects?

Many people find doctors intimidating. They don't feel comfortable or qualified to discuss their medications and, in most cases, don't even understand enough medical jargon to follow what the doctor is saying. To make matters worse, doctors often are rushed and don't have time to provide detailed explanations of how to take a new medication and what to expect when taking it. Poor communication often results in people taking their medication improperly, which can lead to serious problems.

Medication errors happen when people do not know what their new medication is for, how to take it properly, or how to recognize and handle potentially severe side effects.

When your doctor prescribes a new medication, you need to ask four key questions.

1) What is the Name of this drug?
2) What is it Used for?
3) How should I Take it?
4) What are the Side effects?

Remember this: NUTS—Name, Use, Take, and Side effects. Don't leave the doctor's office without asking and understanding the answers to these four questions. Be sure to write down this information so you don't forget.

Your doctor works for you. Don't be afraid to ask questions. Learning which questions to ask can be one of the most important steps to prevent medication errors. It is your right and your responsibility to get the information you need before you take any drug. Your health (and your life) depends on it.

"I'm Giving You an ACE for Your BP"

The doctor told Steve, "Your BP is elevated. It's 142/93. I'm giving you an ACE inhibitor for your hypertension. It's called lisinopril. You are to take 10 mg every day. You'll need to watch your potassium intake and call me if you start to have a dry cough. Any questions?"

Steve just shook his head and said, "No."

What Steve *wanted* to ask was the following:

- What does it mean that my *BP* is *elevated*? Is that bad or does elevated mean it's good?
- What is *hyper* ... something? That sounds bad; am I sick?
- What is the name of the drug? *Lis* ... something?
- When am I supposed to take it? Does "every day" mean every morning or every night or whenever I want to take it?
- What if I *forget* to take it and *miss* a dose?
- Should I take it with food or on an empty stomach?
- Are there any *side effects*?
- Should I limit any of my activities?
- What has *potassium* in it? What does that have to do with anything?
- Why is the doctor telling me to call if I have a *cough*? That doesn't make any sense!

Even though the doctor gave Steve information about the new medication, Steve was confused. He did not know the name of the medication, why he was taking it, how he was supposed to take it, or the side effects.

R𝗑pert Advice

Every time you get a new medication, ask your doctor the following questions:

> ➤ *What is the Name of this drug?* Know both the generic and the brand name of the drug. If you are getting a generic, your pharmacist should type both the brand name and generic name on the prescription label. For example: lisinopril, generic for Zestril.

> ➤ *What is it Used for?* Ask your doctor to write the use, or reason you are taking the drug on the prescription. For example, "Take one tablet every day *for high blood pressure*." This way your pharmacist will type the reason on the prescription label, and you will keep track of your medications more easily.

> ➤ *How should I Take it?* Be sure that you know exactly how to take the medication *before* you leave the doctor's office. Do not act as if you understand if you really don't. Your doctor can't read your mind. Speak up and ask him to repeat the directions.

> Do not try to remember the directions that your doctor gives you in the office. You will forget these instructions by the time you get home. Write down the instructions or have your caregiver write them down so you will know what to do when you get home. Also, your doctor or pharmacist may have printed information on the drug. Ask for a copy.

> ➤ *What are the Side effects of the new medication?* Be sure that your doctor or pharmacist tells you what side effect to expect with a new drug. These may include headache, upset stomach, dizziness, drowsiness, and fatigue. Additionally, ask your doctor or pharmacist what you should do if you have a side effect. Knowing what to expect from a new drug and what to do can prevent serious harm.

Bottom Line

Remember: NUTS

1) What is the Name of this drug?

2) What is it Used for?

3) How should I Take it?

4) What are the Side effects?

Don't worry about being "difficult." If you do not understand why you are being given a drug or how you should take it, ask questions until you understand.

Safety Tip #4
Guessing Is Gambling. Play It
Safe—Keep a Medication List

You've got ten seconds. Can you name your prescription drugs, the dosages, why you take them, and then list your medication allergies? If you can't, don't beat yourself up. Most people would have trouble retrieving all that information from memory, and if you're unconscious, well, as they say in New York, "fahghedaboutit!" Unfortunately, failing to keep a list of your prescription drugs and known allergies with you at all times could be making you vulnerable to a serious medication error.

Keep a medication list that includes all of the prescription drugs you take as well as over-the-counter drugs, vitamins, nutritional supplements, and herbal products. It's one of the most important things you can do to prevent medication errors.

The medication list has a place for you to write in the names of your drugs, how you are taking them, and why you are taking them. It also includes a place to write in the drug side effects and your medication allergies.

Use the medication list when speaking with your doctor. Have him review it with you at each office visit. This is especially important if you see several different doctors. All of your doctors need to know what drugs you are taking and how you are taking them. This will prevent duplicate medications, adverse drug interactions, and allergic reactions.

It's vital to have the medication list handy if you are admitted to the hospital, especially in an emergency. The emergency room doctor needs a complete list of your medications and allergies to treat you safely and effectively in an emergency.

An Ounce of Prevention

Stan was having chest pains. He thought he was having a heart attack. He called his daughter to come and take him to the hospital. Within moments, Stan was admitted to the emergency room and hooked up to a heart monitor.

One of the first things the emergency room (ER) doctor asked Stan was if he was allergic to any medications. Stan knew that he had had a reaction to something a few years ago, but he could not remember what it was. Next, the ER doctor asked Stan what medications he was taking. Stan only knew that he took something for blood pressure and diabetes, but he did not know the names of the drugs. Stan was also taking some other pills, but he could not remember their names either. Stan's daughter had no idea what medications her father was taking or if he was allergic to any drugs.

Based on that limited amount of information, the ER doctor treated Stan for a heart attack. A short time later, Stan's test results came back. Stan was not having a heart attack. The doctor did not know what was wrong. Stan's chest pains persisted. Stan's daughter became worried. "Why can't they figure out what's wrong?"

The doctor asked Stan what he had eaten recently and if he ever suffered from heartburn. Stan looked surprised. He remembered that he had run out of the drug he took for his stomach acid several days ago. "Could this be what caused my chest pain, Doctor?" Stan said. "Heartburn?"

The doctor immediately ordered a drug to treat heartburn, and within a few hours, Stan's chest pain was gone. Stan and his daughter were relieved, and they promised the doctor that they would make a list of Stan's medications and drug allergies, and keep a copy with them at all times.

R𝗑pert Advice

➢ Line up all of your prescription bottles and over-the-counter medications on the table in front of you. You should include vitamins, herbal products, nutritional supplements, and all other meds, as well as creams and ointments, patches, eye drops, eardrops, and nose drops or sprays. Be sure to list medications that you take routinely as well as medications you only take occasionally.

➤ For each medication, read the label and fill in the information from the label on the medication list. Include the date you started taking the drug, the name of the drug, what it's for, how you take it, and any known side effects.

➤ Update the list when dosages change or when you stop or start a new medication.

➤ If you have questions about filling out the medication list, call your pharmacist for help.

➤ Always keep the med list with you. Fold it and keep it in your wallet or purse.

➤ Be sure to give a copy to your spouse, partner, children, and other potential caregivers. You also should carry at all times a med list for anyone in your care, especially if you are the emergency contact.

➤ Take the list with you to all health-care appointments, including those with doctors, dentists, therapists, and others. Doctors are now asking their patients to bring an updated med list with them to their appointments.

➤ You or your caregiver should review the list with your doctor each visit to ensure that the doctor's list matches your list and that you are taking your medications as prescribed.

➤ If your medication list does not match the doctor's list, clear up any differences with your doctor during the office visit.

➤ Make sure you know what medications you are on and how to take them before you leave the doctor's office.

➤ Bring a copy of the list to the pharmacy when you have your prescriptions filled and have the pharmacist review it to make sure your list matches the pharmacy's records. Also, bring your information on medication allergies.

➢ You can keep a medication list in many possible formats, including a piece of paper, portable flash drive, software application for your computer, or app for your smart phone; however, many hospitals and doctor's offices do not accept these drives into their computer systems because of privacy issues and concern about computer viruses.

➢ Keep both a paper copy of your medication list and an electronic copy and update both as often as necessary.

Bottom Line

Create a medication list and keep it with you at all times. The medication list is one of the most important things you can do to prevent a serious medication error.

Bonus

Make your own medication list by using the blank copy in the back of the book. Go to www.drmarysue.com to download a free copy of a blank Medication List.

Safety Tip #5
Keeping It All Together: The Personal Health System

From the doctor's office to the hospital, to the pharmacy, to home, it is up to you to help prevent medication errors. The Personal Health System (PHS) is an ongoing record of your medical history, doctor's visits, hospitalizations, medications, lab tests, and X-rays. The PHS is the tool that will help promote active communication and continuity between you and your doctors and other health-care providers. The PHS is the one source that will help ensure that every one of your doctors has all of the information they need to give you the safest medical care.

What Is a Personal Health System?

A Personal Health System (PHS) is a complete and accurate record of your medical history and current health information. The Personal Health System is a binder with specialized forms that is kept up-to-date by you or your caregiver. The PHS is brought with you to each doctor's appointment to ensure that your doctor has the most up-to-date information about your medications and other aspects of your health care. Keeping all of your health information in one place and bringing it with you to your doctor appointments will help build the important doctor-patient partnership necessary for your medical care.

Your Personal Health System Binder Contains the Following:

- personal information
- emergency contact information

- medical history
- medication list
- medication allergies
- immunization records
- laboratory test results
- surgeries and hospitalizations
- insurance information

The Personal Health System to the Rescue!

Tom didn't look good. He was short of breath and complaining of chest pains. His coworkers decided to call 9-1-1 and get Tom to the hospital. One of Tom's coworkers called Jean, Tom's wife, and told her to meet the ambulance at the hospital. Before she left the house, Jean grabbed Tom's Personal Health System binder. This binder contained all of Tom's important health records as well as his insurance information.

Tom was wheeled into the emergency room (ER). The emergency room doctor wanted to get some information from Tom. He needed to know Tom's health problems as well as any medications Tom was taking. He also needed to know if Tom had allergies to certain medications.

Tom was too weak to provide this information. He was scared, nervous, and confused. He told the doctor that he would have to get this information from his wife. Jean arrived a few minutes later with Tom's Personal Health System binder. Jean handed the binder to the doctor and told him that all of Tom's health information was in there.

The ER doctor opened the PHS binder and saw that Tom had a history of heart trouble. He checked Tom's medication list and saw that he was taking several medications for abnormal heartbeats. He also checked for medication allergies and noted that Tom was allergic to morphine. The information in the Personal Health System gave the doctor enough information to proceed with Tom's treatment very rapidly and safely. It also contributed to Tom's successful and speedy recovery.

R~x~pert Advice

> Keep all of your important medical records, including your medication list and emergency contact information, in a Personal Health System binder.

> Update your Personal Health System and bring it with you every time you see your primary care doctor, specialists, dentist, and therapists.

> Bring your Personal Health System with you to the hospital.

Bottom Line

Keeping important health information in a Personal Health System is the smartest thing you can do to prevent dangerous medication errors from happening to you or someone you care for.

Bonus

Go to www.drmarysue.com to order your own Personal Health System.

Part 2

Your Doctor Is Not a Mind Reader: Preventing Medication Errors at the Doctor's Office

Partner with Your Doctor

There is a new approach to health care called the "doctor-patient" partnership. Your doctor is the medical expert and makes the critical decisions about your health care, but as a "partner," you will actively participate in the decisions that affect your treatment and care.

Becoming a partner with your doctor means that you take the responsibility to prepare for doctor appointments by updating your medication list and other health records as well as bringing along any new information that you get from specialists or other health-care providers. It means that you will keep your doctors informed of any new allergies or side effects that you have had to your medications. It also means that you will follow the advice and instructions your doctor gives you and follow up with him if problems arise after you get home.

Partnering with your doctor is critical to preventing serious medication errors and getting the care you need. Your doctor wants you involved. The more you know about your illnesses and medications, the safer you will be.

Safety Tip #6
Know before You Go! Prepare
for Your Doctor Appointment

As a partner in your health care, your role begins the night before your doctor appointment when you take a few minutes to prepare. This will go a long way in making the most of your doctor's time and getting the care you need. There are two things to do before each doctor appointment.

1) Write down the questions or concerns that you have for your doctor.

2) Update your medication list and other health records.

"Why Are You Here Today?"

Dave did not feel well. He had been having trouble breathing and noticed his ankles were swollen. His wife told him he needed to see his doctor, so she made an appointment for him.

Dave showed up for his appointment twenty minutes late, and the receptionist gave him a form to fill out. The form had questions about his past health issues, medications, allergies, insurance, and other things. Dave did not know the answers to any of these questions. He handed the form back to the receptionist and told her he could not fill it out.

Dave went into the exam room. When the doctor entered, he asked Dave, "Why are you here today?" Dave simply said, "I dunno; my wife made me come." The doctor continued to ask, "Have you been having any problems?" Dave got nervous and forgot about his breathing difficulties and swollen ankles. He just said no.

The doctor began to examine Dave and checked his blood pressure. It was high. The doctor also checked Dave's ankles and noticed they were very swollen. The doctor asked Dave if he had been having trouble breathing or if he had any trouble walking with the swollen ankles. Dave answered yes.

"How are you taking your blood pressure medicines?" the doctor asked.

"One of the pills makes me go to the bathroom a lot, so I stopped taking it a few weeks ago."

The doctor told Dave that not taking that pill for several weeks was what caused his blood pressure to become high and his ankles to swell. He instructed Dave to begin to take his diuretic—or "water pill"—and to check his blood pressure every day. He was to call the doctor back if his blood pressure readings were high. Dave realized that by not taking his medication correctly he had actually caused his own problems today. He knew he needed to take more responsibility for his blood pressure from now on or he could cause some serious problems.

Dave now comes prepared to his doctor's visits with his blood pressure readings and his questions written down so if he becomes nervous and confused he can remember. He also updates his list of medicines and the doses he is taking so his doctor knows exactly how he is taking them. Now Dave remembers to tell his doctor about any bothersome side effects and gets advice on how to handle them. This small amount of preparation helps Dave's doctor take better care of him.

R$_x$pert Advice

➢ Take some time before your next doctor's visit to write down the questions that you would like to discuss with your doctor. This will help to make sure that you do not become confused or forget something important.

➢ Remember to bring the list of questions with you to your appointment and have it handy when you meet with the doctor. Bring a pen, so that you can write down the doctor's answers. Do not try to keep everything in your head. It's too easy to become confused and forget some very important information by the time you get home. If necessary, your caregiver can help ask the doctor questions and help you to understand the answers.

➢ Bring a complete and up-to-date list of your medications to every doctor's appointment to review with your doctor.

➢ Bring your Personal Health System with you to all doctor's appointments to be sure your doctor has all of your important medical information.

Bottom Line

A little bit of preparation goes a long way in preventing medication errors. Take some time before your next doctor's visit to write down your questions and update your medication list.

Bonus

"Questions to Ask Your Doctor" is a preprinted form that you can download free from www.drmarysue.com.

Safety Tip #7
"Med Rec," not "Med Wreck."
Review Your Medication
List with Your Doctor

Medication reconciliation, or "med rec" for short, is a medical term that means you compare your medication list to the list of medications your doctor has on file for you. This way, any differences between your med list and your doctor's list will be cleared up (or reconciled) before you leave the doctor's office.

You can prevent some of the most serious medication errors just by telling your doctor what medications you are taking and exactly how you are taking them. It is very important that you update your medication list including prescriptions, vitamins, laxatives, supplements, over-the-counter drugs, and herbal or natural products and bring it with you to every doctor appointment.

"Med Wreck"

Tom did not feel well. He had a constant headache, he was having trouble catching his breath, and his heart was pounding. He took his blood pressure. It was 163/99. Tom called his doctor and made an appointment for that day.

Tom updated his list of medicines including all of his prescriptions and over-the-counter drugs. He also wrote down his blood pressure readings over the past few days.

Tom went to his appointment prepared. When his doctor asked him why he was there, Tom said, "I haven't been feeling well. I have had a headache and I'm having trouble breathing. I took my blood pressure today. It was 163/99. My blood pressure has been high for the past few days, so I made an appointment to see you."

The doctor asked Tom what medications he was taking, and Tom said, "I have my list right here." The doctor reviewed the list of medications he had on file for Tom and compared it against Tom's list and found several problems.

Tom had not been taking the new blood pressure medication he was prescribed at his last appointment. He had gone to the pharmacy to have it filled, but it was so expensive he decided not to get it. Additionally, Tom had been trying to lose weight and was taking some over-the-counter dietary supplements to help with weight loss. The supplements contained caffeine and weight-loss herbs.

By reviewing Tom's medication list with the list he had in Tom's medical chart, the doctor could see exactly what was wrong. He told Tom that he needed a new blood pressure medication, but gave him a prescription for a generic, less expensive drug that was just as effective. He also told Tom the dietary supplements he was taking had caffeine and herbs that could cause his blood pressure to be high. He told him to stop taking them. Tom was then instructed to get the new blood pressure medication filled and take his blood pressure every day. He was to call the office if his readings were high.

The doctor also advised Tom to check with the pharmacist before taking any over-the-counter drugs or supplements. The pharmacist could check for any dangerous drug interactions.

Tom was glad that he had brought his medication list with him to the doctor's office today. His doctor was able to see what medications he was taking (and what he wasn't taking) and exactly how to help him.

R_xpert Advice

> ➤ Update your medication list and take it with you to every doctor appointment. The list should include prescription medications; topical creams, lotions, gels; patches; syrups; over-the-counter drugs for allergies, upset stomach, and pain; vitamins, herbal products, dietary supplements, and anything else that you are taking or using.

➢ Ask your doctor to review your list at every visit and make sure your list matches his. If your med list does not match your doctor's list, get it straightened out before you leave the office. You should know what medications you are supposed to be taking and exactly how you should be taking them.

➢ You can keep a medication list using applications for your cell phone, portable flash drives, and software applications for your computer or iPad; however, many hospitals and medical offices do not accept these drives into their computer systems due to privacy issues and computer viruses. A simple handwritten list or printout may be your best bet.

Bottom Line

Keep an updated medication list and review it with your doctor at every visit.

Bonus

Go to www.drmarysue.com to download a blank Medication List.

Safety Tip #8
Ignorance Is Not Bliss: Know
Your Medication Allergies

Medication allergies can cause a mild rash, shortness of breath, and may even lead to death. Your doctor absolutely must know if you are allergic to any medications, including antibiotics like penicillin or sulfa; pain medications like morphine or codeine; or over-the-counter drugs like ibuprofen, aspirin, or naproxen.

Symptoms of a drug allergy can include a rash, hives, itchy patches of skin, or sensitivity to sunlight. Other more serious symptoms can include swelling of the face or tongue, difficulty breathing, fever, and muscle or joint aches.

A severe reaction can cause a state known as *anaphylaxis*, meaning a severe potentially fatal allergic response causing difficulty breathing, skin redness, swelling, itching, and fluid buildup. It may also include extremely low blood pressure, lung spasm, and shock.

Most allergy symptoms do not happen the first time you take a drug. The allergic response is much more likely to occur days or weeks after the first dose. If you suspect you are having an allergic reaction, contact your doctor or pharmacist at once.

"He Has a Bad Rash and He's Having Trouble Breathing"

John was a junior in high school. His dentist recommended he have his wisdom teeth removed and gave John's mom the name of an oral surgeon. The wisdom teeth came out without difficulty, and the oral surgeon gave John a prescription for Vicodin to help with the pain. Shortly after arriving home, the anesthesia began to wear off and John's mom gave him the first dose of Vicodin. John felt better, and his mom continued to give John the Vicodin for the rest of the day.

After his third dose of Vicodin, John broke out in a red and itchy rash all over his body. He also started to have trouble breathing. John's mom contacted the oral surgeon who told her that John was having a severe allergic reaction to the Vicodin and to get him to the nearest emergency room fast.

In the ER, the doctor gave John an antihistamine and prednisone to treat the allergic reaction. He was told never to take Vicodin or any other drug containing codeine again.

A few months later, John twisted his knee in a football game. His mom took him to the family doctor to have it checked. The doctor examined John's knee and gave him a prescription for Lorcet to help with the pain. During the office visit, John's mom spoke up. She told the family doctor about the severe allergic reaction John had to Vicodin after his wisdom teeth were pulled. She told him about the rash all over his body and the difficulty he had breathing. She asked the doctor if the new medicine had any Vicodin or codeine in it.

The doctor looked concerned. Lorcet was another name for Vicodin it contained exactly the same drug as Vicodin. Had John taken the Lorcet he surely would have ended up with another trip to the emergency room. The doctor immediately recorded the Vicodin and codeine allergy in John's chart and prescribed a different drug.

Lucky for John, his mom spoke up. Since this allergy surfaced after oral surgery, the family doctor never would have known about it unless John's mom told him. By speaking up and making sure the doctor knew about her son's allergies, she prevented a severe medication error.

R$_x$pert Advice

> ➤ Know your medication allergies. Know the names of the medications and the reaction you had.

> ➤ Communicate your medication allergies to your doctor, pharmacist, and nurse as well as all specialists, dentists, and other health-care providers.

➢ Never assume your doctor has your allergies in your medical record, especially if this is a new allergy. Your doctor may not know about it.

➢ Remind your doctor, specialist, dentist, and other providers at every visit, of your medication allergies. To say, "I just want to remind you that I am allergic to codeine" helps to prevent a medication error from happening to you.

➢ Write your allergies on your medication list. Show the list to your doctor and make sure he has the allergy noted in your record.

➢ Be sure your caregiver has detailed notes on your medication allergies, the allergy symptoms you had, and when you had them.

➢ Be careful when being given a new drug. If you are allergic to a specific drug like penicillin, you may also be allergic to similar drugs, like cephalexin. Inform your doctor, so he or she can prescribe the best treatment for you.

➢ If you are allergic to a particular brand-name drug, for example Percocet, you will not be able to take the generic form of that drug either. Your doctor needs to prescribe a different drug for you.

➢ If your doctor tells you that you are allergic to a certain class of drugs, for example, painkillers that contain codeine or antibiotics that contain penicillin, then you should not have *any* medications that are in that class of drugs. A well-informed doctor will know which drugs to prescribe.

➢ If you have had a severe allergic reaction, you may want to wear a medical-alert bracelet or necklace, with that allergy listed on it. This will help in an emergency if you are unable to communicate your medication allergies.

Bottom Line

Always tell your doctor, nurse, or pharmacist if you are allergic to any medications. This will help prevent a severe medication error from happening to you.

Safety Tip # 9
"Beware: Other Rare but Serious Side Effects May Occur"

We have all heard the long lists of side effects at the end of the drug ads on TV. Some drugs can cause nausea, drowsiness, dizziness, dry mouth, blurred vision, blood disorders, liver problems, kidney problems, headache, ringing in the ears, diarrhea, constipation, fever, fatigue, loss of vision, impotence, hair loss, cough, nervousness, anxiety, and so on.

Most drugs have side effects. A side effect is an unwanted reaction caused by a drug in a particular person and can range from minor (headache or upset stomach) to serious (suicidal urges or bleeding stomach ulcers).

If a side effect is minor, you can usually continue taking the drug until the side effect passes or the course of treatment is complete. If a side effect is severe, call your doctor. He will tell you what to do. You should never stop taking the drug until you have spoken with your doctor first.

"Could Lipitor Be Causing My Muscle Aches?"

Pete had been having some bad muscle pain for a few weeks, and he did not know what was wrong. His muscles felt stiff no matter what he did. He took some acetaminophen, but it didn't help. He thought maybe he was just getting old.

As Pete sat watching TV, a commercial for Lipitor came on the screen. Pete had been taking Lipitor for a few months to lower his cholesterol. At the end of the commercial, the announcer listed all of the potential side effects for Lipitor: muscle pain, stiffness, constipation, diarrhea, fatigue, gas, heartburn, and headache.

Did Pete hear right? Lipitor can cause muscle pain? Could he be having a side effect to the medication? Pete made an appointment to see his doctor.

As Pete suspected, his doctor confirmed that his muscle pain was a side effect of taking Lipitor . His doctor told him that many people have this side effect, and in rare cases, this can progress to a life-threatening muscle breakdown. The doctor took Pete off the Lipitor and put him on a different drug that would not cause the same side effect.

R_xpert Advice

> Ask your doctor and pharmacist if there are any side effects to your medications.

> Read the small sticker on the prescription bottle that tells you what side effects to expect. For example: "May Cause Drowsiness" or "Take with Food to Lessen Stomach Upset."

> Call your doctor if you think you are having a side effect to a drug. The doctor may have you stop the drug and try another one. Never stop taking a drug without talking to your doctor first. Your doctor will give you exact instructions about what to do if you are having a side effect.

> Some side effects, including feeling tired or groggy, happen when you first start taking a drug and may go away over time. Speak to your doctor or pharmacist to make sure the side effects are harmless and to see if you can expect them to go away in time.

> One common side effect, an upset stomach, may improve or go away if you take the drug with food or a snack. Check with your pharmacist to see if this could be the case.

> Sometimes you can reduce the impact of side effects if you take the drug at a certain time of day. For example, niacin causes redness and flushing of the skin. Most people take niacin at bedtime so that they do not

experience this flushing during the day. Other drugs, like antihistamines, can cause drowsiness, and it's safer to take them at bedtime, especially if you are driving or operating heavy machinery.

Bottom Line

Side effects may be serious and you need to speak with your doctor if you suspect you are having a bad side effect. Often you can manage mild ones easily when you have the right information. Speak to your doctor or pharmacist about any side effects you experience.

Safety Tip #10
Making the Most of Your
Time with the Doctor

During the average annual physical, your doctor may have only fifteen to thirty minutes to spend with you. In that time, your doctor will give you a physical exam, review your medications, draw your blood for lab tests, take your blood pressure, give you immunizations, write new prescriptions, and make referrals to other doctors if necessary. This is a lot to do in a very short time, but it's your time, so make the most of it.

To maximize your time with your doctor, come prepared. Write out your questions and update your med list beforehand. Prioritize your questions or problems, starting with the most important first. Learn to ask questions about your medications and other treatments. Include your caregiver in these discussions to ensure you both understand the information.

Betty's Cure-all Remedy for a Miserable Year

Betty was ready for her yearly doctor's appointment. She had written down her problems and updated her med list. She arrived for her visit early and waited patiently for her examination.

Betty had her list of problems out when her doctor came in, and when he asked how she was, Betty replied,

"I've had a miserable year, thank you very much.

My blood pressure is high, and my sex drive is low.

My vision is poor; I drive really slow.

I'm tired all the time; I really can't sleep.,

And that niacin you gave me

Makes my skin start to creep.

I have pain in my back, neck, shoulder, and thigh.

I have so much pain, I just want to sigh.

Some pills make me high,

Some pills make me low.

Am I taking them right?

I really don't know.

But Doc, don't you worry

There's a "cure-all" you see.

Just give me the new drug,

That I saw on TV."

The doctor was so overwhelmed he didn't know where to start to help Betty. He would just have to take it one ailment at a time.

R$_x$pert Advice

- ➤ Before the doctor's visit, use the Doctor's Office Visit form to make a list of questions, concerns, or problems that you want to discuss during the appointment.

- ➤ Keep the appointment on track and get your questions and concerns addressed in order of priority. If you have a long list of issues and ailments, do not be upset if your doctor asks you to come back for a follow-up visit. There may not be time to discuss every issue in one visit.

- ➤ Use a friendly tone of voice and a pleasant manner. Be courteous, respectful, and appreciative of your doctor's time. Avoid confrontational or accusing speech. Be direct, not vague or uncertain. Get right to the point with specific examples of your problem.[9]

➢ Do not pressure your doctor for a new medication. Know that more medication may not be better. Do not pressure your doctor for a drug just because you saw it on television. Your doctor knows your medical history and what is right for you. Taking medications that you do not need can lead to medication errors.

➢ Be honest with your doctor about how you *really* take your prescription medications. Your doctor needs to know if you are not taking your medications as prescribed or if you stopped taking a pill because you ran out, can't afford it, or if you had a bothersome side effect. Your doctor forms your treatment plan on the assumption that you are taking your medications correctly. If you are not, this will make a big difference in your care.

➢ If your doctor asks how much alcohol you consume, be honest and say exactly how much. Alcohol can increase the effects of many drugs and cause serious side effects and drug interaction problems.

➢ Tell your doctor if you are using illicit (street) drugs. This is critical to preventing medication errors and negative drug interactions. Keeping this information from your doctor can be dangerous.

➢ Smoking may affect your drug therapy. Tell your doctor if you are smoking or using tobacco products.

➢ Before you leave the office, review all the information with your doctor or the nurse and write it down so you can remember it after you get home. Be sure to get a callback number in case you have additional questions.

Bottom Line

Prepare for your office visits and ask questions about your medications to make the most of your time with your doctor. Remember, your doctor is there to help you.

Bonus

Go to www.drmarysue.com to download the Doctor's Office Visit Form. This includes a place to write all of your questions and the answers you receive about your new medications.

Safety Tip #11
Saving Face: What to Do if You Are Too Embarrassed to Ask Questions

Certain health issues are just too embarrassing for most people to feel comfortable discussing with their doctor. Sexually transmitted diseases, erectile dysfunction, etc. may be topics you would prefer to avoid entirely; however, your doctor needs to know about these health issues to provide you with the proper treatment. While it may be new or embarrassing for you, your doctor and other providers are very comfortable discussing these issues in a respectful and professional manner. Believe me, you are not the first.

The "Talk"

Bill was ready. He was finally going to ask his doctor for Viagra. He had seen the commercials on TV, and now he was ready to have "the talk." Bill went to see his doctor, and surprise! It was not Dr. Jones who would be seeing him; it was Susie, the nurse practitioner. Susie examined Bill and then asked him if he had any questions or concerns to discuss. Bill was embarrassed, but decided to speak up anyway. He started by telling the nurse practitioner about certain changes in his recent sex life and wondered if taking Viagra would be right for him. Susie reviewed Bill's medical history and ran some blood tests. She told Bill she would prescribe Viagra after the results of the tests were back and she could safely determine if that would be the right treatment for him.

The nurse practitioner handled Bill's issue in a thorough and professional manner. Although he had been embarrassed at first, he was glad he spoke up and got the best care and treatment he needed.

R_xpert Advice

> If you are too embarrassed to bring up certain health issues, use the Questions to Ask Your Doctor form and simply write down your questions and concerns. When your doctor asks if you have any questions, hand over the form and ask him to read it. This is an easy way to begin a discussion.

> Ask your caregiver to bring the embarrassing subject up for you. Having another person there to help ask questions can make it easier to discuss embarrassing issues.

> Never be embarrassed to tell your doctor you don't understand what he is telling you. Medical information is complicated, and most people easily get confused. If you are having a hard time understanding, politely ask your doctor to repeat the information. Do not fear that your doctor will be angry or think less of you. In fact, the doctor wants you to speak up and get the information you need.

> Remember to write down the information as your doctor is giving it to you. Your caregiver can take notes as well. This will help you to remember what your doctor said once you get home.

> If you speak another language, ask if anyone in the office speaks your language and could translate for you. If you have trouble reading, do not be embarrassed. Let the doctor know and ask for easy-to-read, printed materials in your language.

> Do not leave the doctor's office until you understand everything the doctor told you.

Bottom Line

Your doctor is a professional and is accustomed to having delicate conversations. He is bound by confidentiality not to discuss your health concerns with anyone else. Speak up (even if it is embarrassing) and get the answers you need. Your health depends on it.

Safety Tip #12
TV Is No Guide. Don't Pressure Your Doctor for Drugs You Saw on TV

Have you ever pressured your doctor for a new drug you saw on TV? Many people have. In fact, one-fifth of the respondents to a *Consumer's Report* survey said they had asked their doctor for a drug they saw on TV, and nearly 70 percent of the time, their doctor said yes![10]

Drug companies want you to see their ads on TV, then go and tell your doctor what drug you want. Do not fall for this risky sales tactic that is forbidden everywhere else in the world except in the United States and New Zealand. The prescription medications advertised probably are not right for you. Your doctor knows about all the drugs available and which would work best for you.

In 2008, drug companies spent nearly $5 billion on this Direct-to-Consumer (DTC) advertising.[11] Most of the money spent on DTC advertising involved drugs for lifestyle issues such as erectile dysfunction, eyelash length, stomach upset, depression, and insomnia. The drugs advertised, such as Lunesta, Nexium, and Cymbalta, are the newest and often the most expensive drugs on the market. In most cases, these drugs do not represent new treatments. They simply are newer versions of older, less expensive, tried-and-true drugs.

"Siesta": the New Wonder Drug for Sleep

Nancy was having trouble sleeping. She decided that she needed a sleeping pill. Nancy saw an ad on TV for the new drug, Siesta. She wanted to be like the woman in the commercial who looked so happy and well rested.

Nancy made an appointment to see her doctor. She told him that she was having trouble sleeping, and she wanted a prescription for Siesta. She had seen it on TV and thought it would work for her.

Nancy's doctor looked concerned. He knew Nancy and her medical history. He knew that there was no reason for her to have a sleeping pill. Nancy's doctor recommended several non-drug-related alternatives. He suggested that she keep regular sleeping times and get a comfortable bed in a quiet room with the temperature set appropriately. He told her to avoid coffee, tea, or other caffeine-containing drinks before bedtime. He also showed her some relaxation techniques.

Nancy was angry. She told her doctor that she wanted Siesta. She was convinced that it would help her sleep. Nancy's doctor asked her to try the nondrug alternatives first. If these did not work, she could come back and he would start her on a low dose of a sleeping pill that he had a great deal of experience with and had prescribed for many years.

Nancy reluctantly agreed to her doctor's plan and to her surprise, she was able to get some much-needed rest after trying the nondrug alternatives. She learned never to pressure her doctor again and insist that he prescribe a new drug for her. After all, he was the doctor.

R̲xpert Advice

> ➢ Don't fall for drug company advertising. When you see the ads for new drugs on TV, in magazines, or hear them on the radio, realize that this is a sales tactic used by drug companies to up their profits. After seeing the ad, they want you to ask your doctor to prescribe this medication for you. In most cases, this is not the best drug for you.

> ➢ Do not pressure or insist that your doctor prescribe a new drug just because you saw it on TV.

> ➢ If your doctor suggests an older, less expensive drug, try it. Your doctor will know exactly what to expect, it may be just as effective, and you can save some money.

Bottom Line

Your doctor knows your medical condition and will use a familiar drug that will work best for you. Don't pressure your doctor for new, expensive drugs you saw on TV.

Safety Tip #13
Deal or No Deal: Free Drug Samples.
Good Deal or Risky Business?

Everyone likes to get something free. We all like to feel like we are getting a "deal," especially with the high cost of medicines. If you can't afford your medications, drug samples can be a big help, but be careful—free drug samples may end up costing you a lot more money or even causing a deadly mistake.

What You Need to Know before Taking Drug Samples

Drug samples may *not* be a good deal. Samples are a marketing tool designed to increase the sales of new, expensive, brand-name medications. Drug company sales reps give samples to doctors to promote the use of their new drugs. In fact, in 2004, drug companies spent over $16 *billion* in samples, representing one-fourth of their marketing budget.[12]

If your doctor gives you a few samples of a medication that you will be taking for a long time (blood pressure, diabetes, cholesterol, etc.), you may end up paying out-of-pocket for an expensive drug when the samples run out.

Another risk to drug samples is that they may not have clearly written instructions on the package. Your doctor may tell you how to take the sample medication but may not write down the instructions. The instructions you have when you leave his office may be unclear or even forgotten by the time you get home. This may lead to confusion and possibly a medication error.

Adding further risk, drug samples bypass the pharmacist. When the pharmacist fills your prescription, he or she is providing a crucial safety check. The pharmacist is checking for the correct dose, drug interactions, drug allergies, and side effects. Not having this safety check also can lead to medication errors.

In some situations, drug samples *are* a good deal. If you only need a brief treatment (for example: short-term antibiotics or pain relief) and your doctor gives you enough samples to cover the entire length of your treatment, then samples will save you the cost of the drug.

Do the Math

Say your doctor gives you a month's supply of samples for a new brand-name drug to help you lower your cholesterol. It's expected you will be taking this drug for the rest of your life, and it doesn't come in a generic form.

If you have insurance, the brand-name drug will have the highest co-pay. Your co-pay may be $45 per month for that new drug. You have received the first month free in samples from your doctor, so your out-of-pocket cost for the rest of the year ($45 per month x 11 months) is $495.

If you use a generic medication of a similar cholesterol drug, you will have a lower insurance co-payment. Your co-pay may be $15 per month or $180 for a year's worth of medication. The total savings between the new, brand-name drug and the older generic brand is $315.

If you do not have insurance, the out-of-pocket cost for the new cholesterol drug could be prohibitive. For example, a one-month supply of a brand-name cholesterol-lowering drug may cost you $165 *per month* or $1980 per year! You may get the same benefit from a generic drug that costs you $4 per month or $48 per year. Check with your doctor or pharmacist to see if a lower-cost generic drug will give you the same results as the new, more expensive brand-name medication.

R̲xpert Advice

➢ Many drug companies provide doctors with vouchers for new medications instead of the actual pill samples. Ask your doctor to give you a voucher with the new prescription that you can take to the pharmacy to have filled. This way, you will get a prescription bottle with appropriate labeling and directions, and the pharmacist is still in the loop and able to perform a safety check.

➤ If you are currently taking a sample medication, ask your pharmacist to add it to your medication list. Your pharmacist can check to be sure you are taking the correct dose and that there are no medication allergies or possible negative drug interactions.

➤ If your doctor gives you a sample of a new medication, ask him to write down the instructions, including the Name of the drug, why you are Using it, how to Take it, and any Side effects. Remember NUTS to be sure you get all of the necessary information about your new drug.

Bottom Line

Free drug samples may seem like a bargain, but they carry extra risks and you may end up paying more in the long run.

Safety Tip #14
Drug Going Badly: Know
Your Warning Signs

When you get a new prescription, your doctor should tell you exactly which warning signs to watch out for and how to contact him if a problem occurs. Warning signs alert you that something is not right; they should not be ignored.

Knowing the specific warning signs that are unique to you, your illness, and your medications can help prevent problems from occurring and may even save your life.

"Take as Directed"

Maggie was confused. She had two different bottles of warfarin, a blood thinner. Both bottles said, "Take as directed."

At her appointment, Maggie's doctor had told her exactly how to take each one of these pills, but she hadn't understood what he said and she hadn't written it down. Maggie wasn't sure what to do when she got home, so she took one of each pill every day.

A few days later, Maggie noticed new bruises on her arms. She did not want to bother her doctor, so she called her daughter to see if she knew what was wrong.

Maggie's daughter knew exactly what was wrong. She knew that warfarin was a blood thinner and that too much could cause bruises and bleeding. Maggie's daughter realized that her mother had become confused and had taken too much blood thinner, so she called the doctor.

The doctor told her to bring Maggie in immediately. He would need to run a blood test to see how thin Maggie's blood had become. The doctor knew that if he didn't treat Maggie quickly, she would need to be hospitalized.

Maggie was the victim of a medication error. The directions on the bottle—"Take as directed"—did not tell her exactly how to take the drugs, and with no written directions, Maggie had become confused and had guessed what to do.

Maggie's daughter knew that from now on, she would go along with her mother to the doctor appointments. She would write down the important information the doctor was giving her, including directions for her medications and any warning signs that could lead to serious problems.

Rxpert Advice

- ➤ Before you leave the doctor's office, know the warning signs of overdose, allergy, and dangerous side effects.

- ➤ Ask your advocate or caregiver to write down the warning signs. Do not rely on your memory; this is complicated information and easy to forget. Repeat the information back to your doctor to confirm that you understood.

- ➤ Warning signs will alert you that you are having a problem and need to call your doctor. Know whom to contact if you suspect a problem. Know whom to call during regular office hours and at night (the doctor on call) and how to reach them. Be sure to get both your doctor's phone number and the phone number of the doctor on call. Find out beforehand what to do if the number goes to an answering service and you need immediate attention.

- ➤ Never hesitate to call your doctor. If you are having problems, your doctor needs to know right away. Working together with your doctor will help prevent medication errors.

- ➤ If you suspect a life-threatening emergency, call 9-1-1 right away. Do not hesitate. When you get to the emergency room, the ER staff will contact your doctor from there.

Bottom Line

Know the warning signs of various problems that may occur after you get home, and know how to reach your doctor if you need extra care.

Safety Tip #15
Invaluable Help: The Role of the Advocate at the Doctor's Office

What is an "advocate," and why is this person so important?

A health-care advocate is that special person (spouse, adult child, or caring friend) who accompanies you to your doctor's appointments and then helps coordinate your health care after you get home.

Your advocate can help you prepare for your doctor visits by writing down your questions and prioritizing them. Your advocate can also update your medication list.

During the office visit, your advocate can help communicate with your doctor. He or she can ask important questions that you may not think to ask when you are sick or under stress, and then they can write down the doctor's answers.

Another important role of the advocate is to help coordinate your care among different doctors. He or she can help schedule follow-up tests and visits as well as make sure your prescriptions are filled and taken properly. Your advocate should also know the warning signs to watch for and what to do if your condition worsens after you get home.

This person may also be your caregiver. The term *caregiver* usually refers to that person, usually friend or family, who helps an older person with bathing, dressing, feeding, and taking meds on time. A caregiver also provides companionship and social support.

"Sit Down and Don't Say a Word"

My mother lives in Detroit, and I live in Denver. It's hard to know what is really going on with her health from that far away. During a recent visit, I asked if I could come with her to her doctor appointment just to make sure I was clear about her overall health-care and medication plan.

"Well, I guess you can come," she said. "You drive your car, and I'll drive mine." Mom told me her appointment was at 10:00 a.m. and gave me some vague directions.

I left with plenty of time to get there; however, I soon realized the directions Mom had given me were inaccurate. I pulled over and set my GPS for the doctor's address. I arrived right at ten o'clock and looked around the waiting room for my mom. I did not see her, and the receptionist told me that she was already in the exam room. *Hmmm,* I thought. *Is the doctor running early?*

I entered the exam room, and found my mom seated on the exam table looking guilty. "You can't shake me that easily, Mom," I told her. "You ought to know that giving me the wrong directions and telling me the wrong time wouldn't prevent me from being here with you today."

"Sit down and don't say a word," she said.

The doctor entered the room, and I introduced myself. After some friendly conversation, I explained that I would like to take some notes during the exam. He agreed and began to examine my mom. He asked her if she had been having any problems, and she brought out her list. She went through each issue, and I jotted down the doctor's responses. When she got to the third item on the list, she looked apprehensive. "I've been having some chest pains," she said. "They come and go, especially when I get upset." I must have come out of my chair, because she glared at me.

"Chest pains?" the doctor asked. "Why didn't you call me?"

"Because I didn't want to bother you," my mom said. "Besides, they always go away."

"We'll have to do some tests before you leave today," he said and left the exam room.

"Mom," I began, "chest pains? Why didn't you say something?"

"Don't start with me," she said. "It's my health, and I know what I'm doing."

No wonder she didn't want me here today, I thought. *She's having problems and doesn't want me to know.*

The doctor returned and performed an EKG and said that he wanted to schedule a few more tests later that week. He went on to explain the tests and why he wanted them done. He also explained how the blood flowed through the heart and the reasons why he thought Mom was having chest pains. He gave us several warning signs of problems that we should watch for after we got home, and he said he was going to prescribe a new medication.

We asked the doctor the NUTS questions: the name of the new medication, its use, how to take it, and the side effects. The doctor answered the questions and even provided some written information to take home. I wrote down all of the information and then asked him to repeat a few instructions so I was sure I got them right.

Mom and I left the office in an uneasy silence. Finally, Mom spoke. "I'm glad you were here with me today. I don't know what I would have done if it had been really bad news. Thanks for jotting down all of that information. I was too upset to comprehend one word he said, much less write it all down. Maybe you can go over it with me later tonight."

I told her that I would stay with her until all the tests were done and make sure everything was all right. I would also ask my brothers to look in on her more frequently and to accompany her to her doctor's visits.

Mom was unaccustomed to having her children care for her, but at this time in her life, she needed us to care and advocate for her.

R$_x$pert Advice

> ➤ Spend some time with your advocate before your doctor's appointment to write down any questions or concerns that you wish to discuss with your doctor. Ask them in order of priority, and discuss the most critical issues first so you don't run out of time.

➢ Ask your advocate to help you update your medication list. Add all new drugs and take off any that you have stopped taking. Be sure to include over-the-counter drugs, vitamins, and supplements.

➢ Ask your advocate to bring any information from other doctors you have recently seen, including lab test results and X-rays.

➢ During the doctor's appointment, ask your advocate to write down the information he is giving you. Have your advocate repeat the information back to the doctor so you both understand it.

➢ Bring your Personal Health System with you to your doctor's appointments. This will help keep all of your important information in one place.

Bottom Line

Ask your advocate to accompany you to your doctor's appointments. Rely on your advocate to communicate with your doctor effectively and help coordinate your medical care.

Part 3

Go NUTS: Preventing Medication Errors at the Pharmacy

All of us will probably take prescription medications during our lifetime. Some of us will only take a few, while others will take up to fifteen to twenty different medications, not including over-the-counter drugs and natural remedies. Most people think that they can take medications without any guidance, but taking medications correctly isn't as simple as it seems. Studies estimate that nearly half of Americans do not take their medications as directed, causing severe and sometimes fatal medication errors.[13]

The community pharmacist is one of the most trusted and accessible health-care professionals. After years of study, he or she is knowledgeable in prescription drug therapy and is there to help you. However, it is up to you to find the right pharmacist and ask for help. Find a pharmacist who will take the time to explain your medications to you, including complicated dosing instructions and side effects. Your pharmacist should be willing to develop a relationship with you and make you feel comfortable discussing your medications. The pharmacist should also be willing to provide you with recommendations for cost-saving alternative drugs, generic substitutions, and over-the-counter therapies.

Take the time to get to know your pharmacist and learn which questions to ask to get the care you need. Do not leave the pharmacy without knowing exactly what you are taking and why you are taking it. It is up to you to know how to take your medications and if there may be potentially serious side effects. Ask for written information and the pharmacy phone number in case you have questions later. Taking time to develop a relationship with your pharmacist when you are healthy will help you get the care you need when you are ill. Get to know your pharmacist. You'll be glad you did.

Safety Tip #16
Go NUTS! Ask Your
Pharmacist for Help

Asking your doctor the four NUTS questions will provide you will a great deal of information about your new drug. Asking your pharmacist the same four NUTS questions ensures that you understand what your doctor told you, and it provides one of the most critical safety checks in preventing medication errors. Asking the pharmacist to restate the name of the drug, what it is used for, how to take it, and the side effects, confirms the information that your doctor gave you and makes sure you are getting the right drug. So the next time you are at the pharmacy counter and the pharmacist asks you if you have any questions, don't say no. Say "Yes, I do" and ask the four NUTS questions to get the answers you need to take your medications safely.

"Zyrtec or Zyprexa?"

Joe went to see his doctor for his allergies. He felt miserable. He had a runny nose, stuffy head, and watery eyes. Joe's doctor gave him a prescription for Zyrtec to help his allergies. He told Joe to take it once a day and that he should start feeling better in a few days.

Joe went to the pharmacy to have his new prescription filled. The pharmacist filled the prescription and then asked Joe if he had any questions. Joe said, "Yes, this is a new prescription for me. What is the name of the drug?" The pharmacist told Joe that the name of his new drug was Zyprexa. He went on to tell Joe that the drug was used for bipolar disorder and schizophrenia.

Joe was shocked. This was not right. Joe told the pharmacist that the doctor had given him a prescription for Zyrtec. He had been to his doctor for his allergies. He did not have bipolar disorder or schizophrenia! Joe realized that the information the pharmacist was giving him did not match what his doctor had told him. There had been a mistake.

The pharmacist was stunned. He quickly reviewed the prescription and realized that the drug names looked so much alike, that he had mistaken Zyrtec for Zyprexa and had filled the prescription with the wrong drug. Had Joe not asked to review the medication with him, he would have given him the wrong drug.

The pharmacist filled the Zyrtec prescription with the right drug and was thankful the mistake had been caught before a serious problem had occurred.

R$_x$pert Advice

- ➤ Ask your pharmacist to review your new medication with you. Be sure the information your pharmacist gives you matches what the doctor told you. If the information does not match, there may have been a mistake. Ask the pharmacist to clear up anything that does not seem right to you, even if he needs to call your doctor.

- ➤ Ask the Name of your medication, including the brand name and the generic name. Write them down, or ask the pharmacist to write them down for you.

- ➤ Ask what the drug is Used for (or why you are taking this medication). Ask your pharmacist to type the reason for the medication on the prescription label. For example, "Take one tablet daily *for high blood pressure.*" This will help you to remember why you are taking the medication.

- ➤ Ask how to Take the medication correctly. This is essential to preventing a medication error. Verifying the directions with the pharmacist will ensure that you understand exactly how you should take it.

> ➤ Ask what the *Side* effects are and what to do if you have a side effect. Your pharmacist can tell you what side effects to look for and what to do if one happens to you.

> ➤ Ask your pharmacist for written information about your new drug; this will come in handy after you get home.

> ➤ Get the pharmacy phone number if you have additional questions or still do not understand the directions after you get home.

> ➤ If you are too embarrassed to ask questions face-to-face, then call the pharmacist after you get home and speak to him or her over the phone.

> ➤ If you are still unclear about your directions, ask your caregiver or family member to contact the pharmacist, get things cleared up, and provide you with the correct information.

> ➤ If you have a question about your medication, call the pharmacist for help. *Do this before you take the medication.*

Bottom Line

Get to know your pharmacist and begin an essential partnership that will help you take your medications safely and correctly.

Safety Tip #17
Checkin' It Twice: Review Your Med List with Your Pharmacist

To avoid medication errors, take your medication list with you to the pharmacy and review it with your pharmacist every time you have a prescription filled. This is especially important when getting a new prescription filled, because the pharmacist will check to make certain there are no drug duplications, drug interactions, or allergies. Reviewing your med list with your pharmacist provides a critical safety check.

Double Trouble

Andy went to the pharmacy to have a prescription filled. His doctor had prescribed a new blood pressure medicine today because his old blood pressure medication was not doing the trick. Andy handed the prescription to the pharmacist and also gave her a copy of his medication list. He asked the pharmacist to review the list so she could see what medications he was taking and to be sure that he was taking them correctly.

In reviewing the list, the pharmacist saw a problem. The new prescription that Andy brought in today was very similar to the one that he was currently taking for his blood pressure. She asked Andy if the doctor had told him to stop taking the old medication and start taking the new one. Andy did not know. He just assumed that he should take both pills, since his doctor had not told him to stop taking the old one. The pharmacist knew that if Andy took both of these pills together, it could lead to a dangerous drop in blood pressure.

The pharmacist called the doctor to clarify the directions. The doctor wanted Andy to stop the old blood pressure medication and begin taking the new one. The doctor was glad the pharmacist had called him, since he had just assumed that Andy knew to stop taking the old drug.

By reviewing Andy's medication list and checking with the doctor, the pharmacist had avoided a dangerous mistake.

R_xpert Advice

➢ Take your updated medication list to the pharmacy every time you have a prescription filled. Review it with your pharmacist to be sure that list matches the list the pharmacy has on file for you.

➢ By reviewing your current list of medications your pharmacist can

- make sure that your list of medications matches the list on file at the pharmacy,

- review your prescribed dosages with you to be sure that you are taking all of your medications correctly,

- check to be sure that you are not taking two or more drugs that are similar or are doing the same thing,

- make sure that there are no interactions with any of the other prescription drugs you are taking,

- verify that there are no interactions with any over-the-counter drugs, dietary supplements, nutritional products, or herbal remedies you are taking,

- verify there are no interactions with any of the food or beverages you are eating or drinking,

- be sure you are not allergic to any new medications, and

- be sure you have not experienced a bad reaction to the drug or any similar drugs in the past.

Bottom Line

Review your medication list with your pharmacist every time you have a prescription filled. This is especially important when getting new medication.

Safety Tip #18
Read the Prescription Label
Before You Take Your Medicine

Many people assume that they know how to take their meds. They don't even bother to read the prescription label. This can lead to disastrous results. The label contains vital information that will help you take your medications safely and correctly.

Read the label on the prescription bottle (patches, inhalers, eye drops, nasal spray, ointment tube, etc.) *each time* you take your meds. Even if you think that you are certain you know how to take it, read the label. This is a critical safety check and prevents dangerous drug errors.

"I Didn't Even Read the Label"

Ted didn't feel well. He did not know why, but something was wrong. The previous week he had gone to his doctor for his back pain. The doctor gave Ted a prescription for a "pain patch." Ever since, he felt "off" dizzy and sleepy. He almost fell over when he got out of bed in the morning. Ted called his pharmacist to see if this was a normal reaction.

The pharmacist was puzzled, since the patch prescribed for Ted should have worked well for him. Each patch contained a very potent painkiller that was to last for three days. Every three days, Ted was to remove the old patch and put a new one on.

The pharmacist asked Ted how he was using the patch. Ted told the pharmacist that he put a new patch on *every* day, and he left all the old ones on. Right now, he had three pain patches on his back.

Ted had not read the label on the box of patches. He did not know that he was only supposed to apply a new patch every three days and not every day. He had no idea that he was supposed to take the old ones off. By applying a new patch every day and leaving the old ones on, Ted was adding painkiller to his body at more than three times the prescribed rate. No wonder Ted felt weak; he was having a significant drug overdose.

Ted admitted to the pharmacist that he had not read the prescription label on the box. He just assumed he should put a new one on every day. He had never even thought about removing the old ones.

The pharmacist explained exactly how Ted should use the patch, and he instructed him to call the pharmacy with any questions and call his doctor if he was having any more problems. He also told him never to leave the pharmacy without knowing exactly how to take or use his medications.

R_xpert Advice

- ➢ Don't assume that you already know how to take or use your medications. Read the labels and follow the directions every time you take your pills, use an inhaler, or apply a patch. If you do not understand, call your pharmacist and ask for help *before you take or use the medication.*

- ➢ Even if you think that you are taking the medication correctly, you may not be. Ask your pharmacist to review the directions with you just to be sure that you are taking them the right way.

- ➢ Ask the pharmacist if there is a specific time that is best to take it. Ask if you should take it with food or on an empty stomach.

- ➢ Write down what the pharmacist says or ask for written information about your new drug that you can read at home.

- ➢ Add any new medications to your medication list and schedule.

➢ Keep your pharmacist's name and pharmacy phone number handy in case you have questions later.

➢ Always review your new medication with your pharmacist before you leave the pharmacy.

Bottom Line

Never assume you know how to take your medications. Read the prescription label every time your take your meds. This provides a critical safety check.

Safety Tip #19
Deciphering the Directions

As a pharmacist, I have never met anyone who did not have questions about how to take their medications. Even the simple direction, "Take one tablet by mouth twice a day" can elicit a whole host of questions. These include the following, among many others:

- Do I have to take it at the same time every day?
- Do I take it with food or on an empty stomach?
- Should I take it in the morning or at night?
- Should I take it before meals or after meals?
- What should I do if I forget to take it?
- Can I stop taking it when I start feeling better?

Let's face it. Prescription directions are confusing. Most people have questions about how to take their medications correctly. A big part of what the pharmacist does is answering these questions for you. Your pharmacist is there to help and expects you to have questions about your medications. So, when the pharmacist asks if you have any questions, say, "*Yes, I do*," and be sure to get the answers you need.

What Does "Twice a Day" Mean?

At a recent seminar, I randomly picked six members of the audience and asked what the phrase "take one tablet twice a day" meant to them. I received these answers:

- "I take one tablet when I get up and one tablet when I go to bed."
- "I take one tablet at 8:00 a.m. and one tablet at 8:00 p.m."
- "I take one tablet whenever I remember in the morning and whenever I remember at night."
- "I take one tablet at breakfast and one tablet at supper."
- "I take one tablet in the morning and one tablet in the afternoon."
- "I take one tablet twice a day—sometimes during the day, but only if I remember."

As you can see, even with what appear to be simple directions, there are many ways to interpret them. Everyone in the seminar was surprised that there could be so many different interpretations of the same directions.

None of these interpretations is completely wrong. However, depending on the drug, some ways of taking it may be more effective. For example, if the directions say, "take one tablet by mouth twice a day," the drug may be most effective and provide the most coverage if taken every twelve hours. On the other hand, if upset stomach is a common side effect, you may rather take your medication after meals so you have some food in your stomach. If you ask, your pharmacist will tell you the most effective way to take your specific medication.

R$_x$pert Advice

➢ Ask your pharmacist exactly how to take your prescription medications, and be sure that you understand these directions before leaving the pharmacy.

➢ Ask what time of day is best to take your meds and if you need to take them at the same time every day. For example, if a drug will make you drowsy, it is best to take that before bed.

➤ Ask if you should take your medication with food or on an empty stomach. Ask if it will upset your stomach and what you should do if that happens.

➤ Ask if there are any special precautions to take while taking this medication, like avoiding alcohol or not driving a car.

➤ Ask what you should do if you miss a dose or mistakenly double up.

➤ Ask what you should do if you think you are having an allergic reaction. This may include rash, swelling or difficulty breathing.

➤ Ask what the side effects are, like upset stomach, headache or drowsiness, and what you should do if you have side effects.

➤ Ask the pharmacist to thoroughly explain the directions to you. Write these directions down if you need to or ask for written materials to take home.

➤ If you get home and you become confused or forget what the pharmacist told you, call the pharmacist back and get the directions straight *before* you take your meds.

Below is a list of common prescription directions and what they mean. Use this overview to guide you in taking your medication correctly. If you still have questions, ask your pharmacist for help.

Common Prescription Directions:

Q: *What does "Take one tablet by mouth once a day" or "Take one tablet by mouth daily" mean?*

A: Take one tablet once a day, at the same time every day.

Q: *What does "Take one tablet by mouth twice a day" mean?*

A: Take one tablet two times a day, during the hours you are awake, approximately twelve hours apart. Take these at approximately the same time each day. For example, take one pill at 8:00 a.m. and one pill at 8:00 p.m.

Q: *What does "Take one tablet by mouth three times a day" mean?*

A: Take one tablet three times a day, during the hours you are awake, approximately eight hours apart. Try to take these at the same time each day. For example, take one pill at 7:00 a.m., take one pill at 3:00 p.m., and take one pill at 11:00 p.m. (or at bedtime if you go to sleep before 11:00 p.m.).

Q: *What does "Take one tablet by mouth four times a day" mean?*

A: Take one tablet four times a day, during the hours you are awake, approximately six hours apart. Take these at the same time each day. For example, if you wake up at 6:00 a.m. and go to bed at 11:00 p.m., you will be taking four doses of medication during the time you are awake. Space the doses out evenly over the entire day (6:00 a.m., 12 noon, 6:00 p.m., and 11:00 p.m.).

Q: *What does "Take one to two tablets by mouth every four to six hours as needed" mean?*

A: These prescription directions provide you with some flexibility in your dosing schedule depending on how often you need to take the medication. You can take one tablet every six hours when needed (the least amount) or take up to two tablets every four hours when needed (the maximum amount). It also means that you may not need to take any at all! For example, if the prescription label reads, "Take one to two tablets every 4 to 6 hours as needed for pain," you may need to take two pills every four hours when the pain is severe. When the pain lessens, you can decrease the dose to one tablet every six hours, only when you need it.

Bottom Line

Prescription directions can be confusing. Ask your pharmacist to explain the directions to you and be sure you understand exactly how to take the medication before you leave the pharmacy.

Bonus:

Go to www.drmarysue.com for additional prescription directions and what they mean.

Safety Tip #20
Lost in Translation: Language Barriers to Vital Drug Information

If you are one of the twenty-three million Americans who have limited understanding of the English language, this safety tip is for you.

Language barriers to medical information (prescription labels, medication sheets, and verbal communication with the doctor and pharmacist) are a major problem for people who have limited grasp of the English language.[14]

Some pharmacies use non-English prescription labels, especially in areas with a high number of non-English-speaking patients. However, many pharmacies do not provide information to non-English-speaking patients. They rely on the patient's bilingual family or friends to translate the information. Often, important instructions are lost in translation with serious consequences, especially when the patient is responsible for managing his or her own complicated medication regimens.

Lost in Translation
A young Hispanic couple brought in a prescription for their baby daughter to the pharmacy where Jane, the pharmacist was working. The baby was very sick and needed a strong antibiotic for her ear infection. The prescription was for amoxicillin liquid, and the parents were to give 2.5 ml by mouth three times daily, around the clock.

Jane knew the directions were confusing, and she needed to counsel the parents on how to give this drug correctly. The baby's health depended on it. However, she also could tell that the parents spoke little English.

Jane included written information with the medication and dispensed an oral medicine dropper so the parents would be sure to give the right dose, but she still wanted to be sure that the parents understood what to do.

Jane came to the pharmacy counter and told the young couple that she wanted to speak to them about the baby's medication. The couple looked confused and told Jane that they did not speak any English. Jane understood and told the couple that she would be right back. Jane went to the computer and printed out the information about the drug in Spanish. This information told the parents the name of the drug, what it was for, and exactly how it should be given to their daughter. It also gave instructions for properly storing the medication in the refrigerator. The instructions included giving the medication until it was gone and not to stop the drug early, even if the baby looked like she was getting better.

The parents were grateful for the information that was given to them in Spanish and appreciated the printed information that they could take home for a guide. They knew without it, they would never have given the medication correctly and their baby daughter would have suffered as a result.

Rxpert Advice

➤ If you have difficulty speaking or understanding English, ask your pharmacist for help. You have the right to counseling by a pharmacist each time you pick up a prescription. Just to be safe, take someone with you to the pharmacy that can help translate the prescription information for you, or ask the pharmacist if there is someone in the pharmacy who speaks your language and can translate the information for you.

➤ If you request it, the pharmacist may be able to provide printed material about your new drug in your language, so that you can read it when you get home.

➤ If a computer program is used to translate the prescription information from English to another language, check the label carefully; there may be errors in translation.

> ➤ Be sure that you understand all of the directions before you leave the pharmacy.

> ➤ Make sure that you open the bag and verify that the name on the prescription is yours, especially if you have a common last name.

Bottom Line

If you have a limited grasp of the English language, be sure to ask for a translation of the prescription directions in your language. Do not leave the pharmacy until you completely understand the information. This is your right and may even save your life.

Safety Tip #21
Levothyroxine, Metoprolol, and Hydrochlorothiazide— Easy for You to Say

When drugs are brand-new, they have easy, catchy names, like Zocor, Zestril, and Synthroid. However, when drugs go off patent and become available as a generic, they use their generic or chemical names. These names are long, difficult to pronounce, hard to remember, and troublesome to spell. Zocor, Zestril, and Synthroid, are now simvastatin, lisinopril, and levothyroxine sodium. This can be confusing and lead to serious drug errors.

The most significant problem that results from confusion over brand and generic names is the potential to unknowingly take both the brand and generic form of the same drug at the same time. Errors happen when a prescription is originally filled with the brand name and then later on refilled with the generic. It is easy to understand why errors happen, because the pills don't look anything alike and the names are completely different.

"How Was He Supposed to Know They Were the Same Thing?"

Tammy stopped by the pharmacy to pick up her dad, Frank's, prescription refills. The pharmacist explained to Tammy that he had filled one of her dad's medications, Toprol XL with a generic. This would save him some money, and it was the same thing.

Tammy dropped off the bag of meds at her dad's house and told him that she was able to save some money by getting the generic of one of his pills. The bottle was labeled "metoprolol succinate extended-release" and Frank added it to the other pills in his weekly med box. A few days later, Frank felt lousy; he was dizzy and sleepy all the time. He was so lightheaded that he almost fell over when he stood up. Something was not right. He called the doctor, who told him to come in and bring all of his medications with him.

On reviewing Frank's meds, the doctor realized what was wrong. Frank had two bottles of his blood pressure medication. One was the brand name, Toprol XL and the other was the generic, metoprolol succinate extended-release. Frank had added the generic to his pillbox and had unknowingly been taking both the brand-name pill and the generic pill of the same drug. He had not realized that he had been taking twice the amount of blood pressure medication than he should have been. This was causing his blood pressure to drop dangerously low. The doctor explained this to Frank and told him exactly how to take his medication.

Frank was glad nothing was seriously wrong with him, but he was genuinely perplexed as to how this could have happened. The two drugs that were the exact same thing did not look anything alike. They did not have the same names; in fact, the names were very different. How was he supposed to know that Toprol XL and metoprolol succinate extended-release was the same thing? Frank realized that taking his medications correctly was not an easy thing to do. From now on, he would make sure he asked his pharmacist to explain the brand name and the generic names to him and to show him what they looked like. He never wanted to make that mistake again.

R$_x$pert Advice

> ➤ Ask your pharmacist to tell you the brand name and the generic names of all of the drugs you are taking. Write both drug names on your medication list so that you don't forget or become confused when you get home.

> ➤ Knowing both the brand name and the generic names of your drugs can help prevent mistakes. Taking both the brand and the generic form of the same drug at the same time is a severe error and happens more often than you may think.

➤ Ask your pharmacist to help you write down the names of your drugs on your medication list. If necessary, ask your pharmacist how to spell and pronounce the long drug names.

➤ If necessary, ask your pharmacist to review your medication bottles with you. Ask the pharmacist to go over each one with you to be sure that you are not taking two (or more) of the same drug at the same time by mistake.

➤ If you are the advocate or caregiver for an elderly parent or spouse and you are confused by all the pill bottles that accumulate over time, ask your pharmacist to go over these with you. Get rid of any bottles that you don't need. Keeping old or unused medications lying around the house only leads to confusion and possible mistakes.

Bottom Line

Know both the brand and the generic names of your drugs. Write these names on your med list to help prevent serious mistakes.

Bonus

Go to www.drmarysue.com for the brand and generic names of fifty commonly prescribed medications.

Safety Tip #22
Brand Name v. Generic:
What's the Difference?

Many people ask me, "Are generic drugs the same as brand-name drugs?" The differences between brand-name and generic drugs are usually minimal, but many people say they react differently to generics and are hesitant to try them.

The main chemicals (drug) in the brand name and generic are the same. The difference is in the fillers and binders that make up the rest of the tablet. These may cause more or less of the drug to be released over a certain period, so you may, in fact, have a different effect from the generic form of the drug. In some instances, people have had an allergic reaction to the fillers and binders in the generic product when they could take the brand name just fine.

"I'm Allergic to Generics"

George didn't trust generic drugs. On one occasion, he had developed a bad rash after his pharmacist had given him a generic form of penicillin, and from then on, he only took brand names. He told the pharmacist, "I'm allergic to generics. Fill my prescriptions with brand names only."

The pharmacist thought George's allergy was due to the penicillin itself and not the generic form, but he understood George's concern and began to fill his prescriptions with brand names only.

The first prescription was for 30 tablets of Norvasc 10 mg at a cost of $95.69 per month. The generic form, amlodipine, cost $4 per month.

The second prescription was for 30 tablets of Synthroid 0.1mg at a cost of $31.69 per month. The generic, levothyroxine, cost $4 per month.

The third prescription was for 30 tablets of Celexa 20 mg at a cost of $156.70 per month. The generic, citalopram, cost $4 per month.

Overall, George was spending $284.08 for three prescriptions every month. This would add up to $3,408.96 every year.

The pharmacist explained the cost difference to George. The generics would cost him a total of $12 per month or $144 per year. He suggested that George try a week's supply of one of the generic drugs to see if he had an allergic reaction. The pharmacist told George that if he had a problem, he could go back to taking the brand-name drug.

George agreed to the trial—after all, $284.08 every month was a lot of money. After a week, George contacted the pharmacist and told him that he was taking the generics without any problems. From now on, he would ask his pharmacist if the generic form of any of new medication was safe and effective for him to use.

Rxpert Advice

➢ Ask your pharmacist if it is safe and effective for you to take the generic medications. Your pharmacist will tell you if it is safe to do so.

➢ Certain brand-name drugs like blood thinners, seizure medications, and diabetes medications, should only be switched to generics under a doctor's watchful eye. You may require additional monitoring to be sure you are getting the same effect from the generic that you did from the brand name. This does not mean that you cannot switch to the generic drug; it just means that your doctor may need to monitor you to be sure that you are getting the same effect.

➢ Several different manufacturers produce generic forms of brand-name drugs. Each manufacturer may produce the drug in a different color or tablet size, so your pills may look completely different from one refill to the next. If you receive a refill of a prescription and the pill looks different from the last one that you took, call the pharmacy to verify that you have the correct drug. Always check with the pharmacist *before you take any of the medication.*

Bottom Line

Check with your pharmacist to see if a generic drug is right for you. Make it a habit to open your pill bottles when you are at the pharmacy. Check to see if the pills in the bottles are the same pills that you received in the past. If not, then make sure to ask the pharmacist if this is the right drug,

Safety Tip #23
SALAD: Sound-*alike*/*Look-**alike** D*rug Names

One of the most common and potentially dangerous medication errors is the mix-up of two drugs that sound alike when spoken or look alike when written. More than 1,500 drugs have names so similar that it has caused them to be confused with other drugs.[15]

Drug companies attempt to come up with new drug names that don't look like or sound like other names. However, new drugs with names that sound remarkably similar to other drugs enter the market all the time. The confusion results in people getting a completely different drug than the one their doctor prescribed.

Arthritis or Depression?

Sheila's arthritis pain was getting worse. She went to her doctor for help. The doctor wrote a prescription for Celebrex, a drug he had prescribed for many years with great success. He was sure this would help Sheila's arthritis pain.

Sheila took the prescription to the pharmacy to have it filled. The pharmacist could not read the prescription. He could not make out if it was Celebrex for arthritis or Celexa for depression. The two drug names looked so similar in the doctor's handwriting that it was nearly impossible to tell them apart. However, these were two completely different drugs.

The pharmacist contacted the doctor, who told him the intended drug was Celebrex. The pharmacist suggested to the doctor that he write the reason for the drug "for arthritis pain" on any future prescriptions to prevent serious drug mix-up errors from happening.

The pharmacist reviewed the new drug with Sheila. He told her the name of the drug was Celebrex and that it was used to treat arthritis pain. The pharmacist also reviewed the prescription directions and any possible side effects she may experience. Sheila was grateful for the advice and left the pharmacy knowing she had the right drug and all the information she needed to take it safely.

R_xpert Advice

➤ Ask your doctor the name of any new drug you are being given and confirm this with your pharmacist when your prescription is filled.

➤ Ask your doctor why you are being prescribed a new drug and confirm this with your pharmacist when your prescription is filled.

➤ Ask your doctor to write the reason you are being given a new medication on the prescription. This way, your pharmacist will type the reason on the prescription label. For example, "for high blood pressure," "for diabetes," "for cholesterol," etc.

➤ Having the reason on the prescription label helps you to remember what the drug is for after you get home.

➤ Add the new drug name and the reason you are taking it to your medication list.

Bottom Line

Prevent drug mix-ups Ask your doctor to write the reason for the drug on the prescription and have the pharmacist type the reason on your prescription label.

Bonus

Go to www.drmarysue.com for a list of thirty commonly used sound-alike/look-alike drugs.

Safety Tip #24
What You Don't Know, Can Hurt You: Preventing Drug Interactions

The effect a drug has on you may not be the one that is intended. This may be due to mixing two or more drugs and having a "drug interaction."

Drug interactions include the following:

➢ taking two drugs that do the same thing and increase the drug's effect

➢ taking two drugs that work against each other and reduce the drug's effect

➢ taking two drugs that change the way a drug works in your body and may increase or decrease its effect

Drug interactions can happen with prescription drugs, over-the-counter drugs, supplements, herbal products, and others. If you discuss all medications that you are taking with your doctor and pharmacist, you can prevent harmful drug interactions.

Alert—Drug Interaction!

Finals week was approaching on campus, and Stacy was fighting a horrible cold. She was coughing, sneezing, and having trouble breathing. She called her parents to see what she should do.

Stacy's mom told her to go to the campus clinic for a prescription. It sounded like she had an upper respiratory infection. Stacy went to the clinic the next day and was given a prescription for amoxicillin, an antibiotic for her chest infection.

Stacy went to the pharmacy where she had all of her prescriptions filled. The pharmacist filled the amoxicillin and asked Stacy to speak with her about her medications. The pharmacist was alerted to a drug interaction with two of Stacy's meds by the pharmacy computer system. The computer alerted the pharmacist that amoxicillin could interact with Stacy's birth control pills and lessen their effect. Stacy would be at risk of becoming pregnant while she was taking the amoxicillin and for at least a week after she had finished it. The pharmacist advised Stacy to use a second form of birth control while she was taking the amoxicillin and for the week following. The pharmacist also told Stacy that if she had any unusual bleeding, she should call her doctor immediately.

Stacy had no idea that amoxicillin could interact with her birth control pills. She was glad the pharmacist had caught the interaction and was able to tell her what to do. She was also glad that she had all of her prescriptions filled at one pharmacy. This allowed her pharmacist to check for interactions with all of her other meds and prevent a dangerous drug interaction from ever happening to her.

R_xpert Advice

> Have all of your prescriptions filled at one pharmacy and be sure the pharmacy has a computer system that automatically checks for drug interactions. Your pharmacist should have a complete list of all of your medications in the computer and will do a check for drug interactions each time you have a prescription filled.

> Keep an updated list of all of your medications and review it with your doctor at every visit to make sure you are not taking two drugs that could interact with each other. This is especially important if you see more than one doctor who prescribes medications for you.

> Review your medication list with your pharmacist every time you have a prescription filled. This is especially true if you have prescriptions filled at more than one pharmacy. The pharmacist should check to be sure there are no drug interactions with any of your other meds.

➤ Ask your pharmacist if there are any over-the-counter drugs, vitamins, laxatives, pain relievers, stomach upset, nutritional supplements, or herbal remedies you should avoid due to possible drug interactions with your prescription medicines.

➤ Read the prescription label, especially the warning stickers that are on the bottle. These stickers may provide information on drug and food interactions.

Bottom Line

Prevent drug interactions by making sure that your doctors and pharmacists know all of the medications you are taking and how you are taking them. This includes prescription and over-the-counter drugs. Contact your doctor right away if you have any unusual symptoms that may be due to a drug interaction.

Bonus

Go to www.drmarysue.com for a list of common prescription drug and herbal product interactions.

Safety Tip #25
Can I Drink Grapefruit Juice?
How to Prevent Serious
Drug/Food Interactions

It's not just other drugs that can cause medication interactions; some of the foods you eat can react badly with your prescription medications. Some foods can cause "drug/food interactions" and may lead to potentially dangerous problems. The food you eat can reduce the amount of drug that enters your body. For example, milk can reduce the amount of the antibiotic tetracycline that enters your body and lessen the effect of the drug.

The food you eat can also increase the amount of drug in your body. For example, grapefruit juice can increase the potency of several medications including "statins" for cholesterol and amiodarone (Cordarone) for heart arrhythmias. Don't take these drug/food interactions lightly. They can lead to potentially serious health problems.

Close Call

Marilyn had high cholesterol. Her doctor gave her a prescription for Zocor (simvastatin) to help lower the cholesterol and told her that losing a few pounds would help as well. Marilyn started taking the Zocor, and a few weeks later decided to start the grapefruit diet. She ate grapefruit for breakfast, lunch, and dinner and drank grapefruit juice in between. She just knew that she would start losing weight and her cholesterol problems would be solved.

A few days into the diet, she started to feel achy. Her muscles felt tired and weak; she had never felt like this before. Marilyn did not know what was wrong, so she called her doctor for help.

The doctor asked Marilyn about the drugs she was taking and exactly how she was taking them. She told the doctor that she had started taking the Zocor and that she had even started the grapefruit diet to lose some weight. Immediately, the doctor suspected the cause of the muscle aches. The doctor told Marilyn that the grapefruit juice was causing a drug/food interaction. It caused the Zocor to accumulate to dangerously high levels in her body, causing muscle aches and pain. This combination was also known to cause serious muscle damage.

The doctor told Marilyn to stop eating grapefruit and grapefruit juice, and he prescribed a different medication for her cholesterol. This was a close call. Marilyn had narrowly escaped a serious problem caused by this interaction. From now on, whenever Marilyn got a new prescription, she would ask her pharmacist if there were any foods she should avoid. She did not want anything like this to happen to her again.

R̽pert Advice

> ➤ Ask your pharmacist if grapefruit juice or other citrus fruits might affect any of your medications. You may need to eliminate grapefruit and grapefruit juice from your diet. Taking your medication at different times than grapefruit juice does not stop the interaction from happening.

> ➤ The good news is that orange juice does not interact with medications the same way that grapefruit juice does. There is no reason to remove orange juice from your diet.

> ➤ Coumadin (warfarin) is a blood thinner and affected by foods that are high in vitamin K. These foods include green leafy vegetables, broccoli, brussels sprouts, spinach, and kale. These foods can decrease

the effectiveness of the blood thinner and may lead to dangerous blood clots. You should eat these foods in limited quantities and the daily amount should remain constant.

➤ Tetracycline is an antibiotic affected by milk and other dairy products. Diary products decrease the amount of tetracycline that goes into your body, greatly reducing the drug's effect. You should take tetracycline one hour before or two hours after eating.

➤ Drugs used to slow or reduce bone loss, like Fosamax, Boniva, and Actonel, are especially affected by food. Any food, even orange juice, coffee, or mineral water can reduce the effectiveness of these drugs. Take these drugs with water only, at least thirty minutes to one hour before the first food of the day.

➤ MAO Inhibitors (monoamine oxidase inhibitors) include phenelzine (Nardil), isocarboxazid (Marplan), and tranylcypromine (Parnate), and are used to treat depression. Other MAO Inhibitors are selegiline (Eldepryl), rasagiline (Azilect), and linezolid (Zyvox). Taking certain foods while taking these drugs can lead to severe headache and a potentially fatal increase in blood pressure (hypertensive crisis). Foods to avoid when taking MAO Inhibitors include those high in tyramine; these include many cheeses, such as American processed, cheddar, blue, Brie, mozzarella, and Parmesan; yogurt; sour cream; cured meats (sausage, salami); liver; dried fish; caviar; avocados; bananas; yeast extracts; raisins; sauerkraut; soy sauce; fava beans; red wine; certain beers; and products containing caffeine, including coffee and chocolate.

➤ Read the prescription label and all of the additional warning labels on the bottle, including stickers that read, "Take on an empty stomach," "Take with food," "Take with plenty of water," "Do not drink alcoholic beverages," etc. If you do not understand the directions or the warning labels, ask your pharmacist before you take the drug.

➢ Take your medications with a full glass of water.

➢ Unless told otherwise by your doctor or pharmacist, do not crush tablets and stir them into your food or liquids. Also, do not take capsules apart and stir them into food or liquids. This may change the way a drug works.

➢ Do not mix medications into hot drinks. The heat from the drink can change the effectiveness of the drug.

➢ Do not take medications with alcoholic beverages.

Bottom Line

Prevent serious drug/food interactions. Ask your pharmacist if you should avoid any foods when taking certain drugs.

Bonus

Go to www.drmarysue.com for a list of drugs that are not to be taken with grapefruit juice.

Safety Tip #26
A Prescription for Disaster:
Mixing Drugs with Alcohol

Mixing alcohol with your medications, whether it is prescription or over-the-counter drugs, is extremely dangerous. Alcohol can make you drowsy, dizzy, and lightheaded, and can increase the effects of certain drugs. Drinking even small amounts of alcohol while taking certain drugs like painkillers or sleeping pills can lead to serious harm. Be smart and do not drink alcohol when taking medications.

"He Only Had a Few Beers"

Daniel had hay fever. His eyes were itchy and his nose was runny. He took his over-the-counter allergy medicine, chlorpheniramine, to help with the symptoms. A few hours later, Daniel was feeling better. He decided to go out with his friends for a few beers. Before he left, he took another allergy pill just to be sure his symptoms didn't come back.

Daniel never had a problem drinking just a few beers before, but tonight was different. Something didn't seem right. He was drowsy, dizzy, and almost fell over when he stood up. His friends were confused—why was Daniel so drunk? He only had a few beers. His friends took him home to sleep it off.

The next day, Daniel was still confused. What had happened? Why had he become so drunk so fast? Then it became clear. The alcohol must have mixed with his allergy pill to cause him to be dizzy and disoriented. He never would have thought that having a few beers while taking an over-the-counter allergy pill would have such a dangerous effect on him. He had been so affected by the combination of his allergy pill and alcohol that his friends took his keys away from him and brought him home. They knew that he was too impaired to drive. Daniel was grateful that his friends had taken care of him. However, he knew from now on that there was no drinking (not even a few beers) while taking any of his medications. There was too much to risk.

R_xpert Advice

> Read the label on the prescription bottle. If there is a sticker (auxiliary label) that warns against drinking, such as "Do Not Drink Alcohol" then do not drink while taking this medication. It could be very dangerous.

> Read the label on the over-the-counter package. If there is a warning about drinking alcohol while taking that medication, then don't drink.

> Drinking alcohol while taking certain medications can make you dizzy, drowsy, or lightheaded. Even small amounts of alcohol with certain medications can make it very dangerous to drive (not to mention against the law).

> Some over-the-counter medications, like those for allergy symptoms, cough, cold products, and sleep aids may contain several different ingredients that each could interact with alcohol. Certain allergy meds or cough-and-cold products may contain up to 10 percent alcohol. Avoid alcohol when taking these products.

> Women are at a greater danger for alcohol-related problems than men. Alcohol is more concentrated in a woman's body and could lead to more harmful effects.

> Older people are at a higher risk for harmful alcohol-medication interactions. As we age, the body's ability to break down alcohol decreases and the alcohol stays in the body longer, increasing the harmful effects. Mixing alcohol with certain medications can lead to serious falls, especially in older people.

➢ Alcohol and medications still interact, even if they are not taken at the same time.

Bottom Line

Do not drink alcohol if you are taking prescription or over-the-counter medications.

Bonus

Go to www.drmarysue.com for a list of medications that are especially dangerous if you drink alcohol.

Safety Tip #27
Secrets to Saving Money on Prescription Medications

As a pharmacist, I have known many people who simply could not afford to pay for their medications. Some people will change the way they are supposed to take their meds; for example, taking a pill every few days, instead of the prescribed once-a-day dose. Some people skip doses, or just stop taking their pills all together. Changing the way you take your medications or stopping your meds to save money is a very dangerous thing to do. Your pharmacist may have some suggestions to help you safely save money and afford your prescription medications.

"I Can't Even Afford a Free Meal"

Joe's doctor was confused. According to Joe's medical chart, he was taking five different drugs. These were for arthritis, high cholesterol, diabetes, depression, and heartburn. However, when Joe was in his office that day for a checkup, his cholesterol and blood sugar were high, he was complaining of arthritis pain, and his acid reflux had gotten worse.

The doctor asked Joe if he was taking all of his medications as prescribed. Joe said, "Oh yes, I take all of my medications every day, just like I'm supposed to."

Joe was secretly thinking, *Doc, the total bill for those five drugs is nearly $1,000 every month! There is no way that I can afford that. I am on a fixed income and my insurance doesn't cover drugs. Right now, I can't even afford a free meal. I haven't taken any medication for the past two months, and I'm afraid something bad is going to happen to me.*

The doctor thought that the medications Joe was taking were not working. He changed some of the drugs and increased the dose of the others. Joe went home with his new prescriptions. He did not even stop at the pharmacy. Why bother? He couldn't afford the new drugs any more than the old.

A few weeks later, Joe went to the emergency room (ER). His blood sugar had become so high he was nauseated and was having trouble breathing. The doctor in the emergency room treated Joe for high blood sugar and asked him what medication he was taking. Joe told the ER doctor that he had stopped taking his medications several months ago because he could not afford them. The ER doctor gave Joe a supply of medication and told him to see his doctor in the next few days.

When Joe saw his doctor, he admitted that he had stopped taking his medications. He simply could not afford them. The doctor reviewed Joe's medications and substituted low-cost generic medications for the high-cost brand-name drugs he had originally prescribed. The doctor also told Joe to ask the pharmacist about the discount drug programs that would bring the cost of these drugs down to as low as $4 a month for each prescription.

Joe took the prescriptions to the pharmacy. The pharmacist was able to fill them with the low-cost generic drugs that were on the $4 drug list. The total bill for an entire month's supply of medication was just $20!

Joe was pleasantly surprised and very relieved. He could finally afford his medications and would take them as prescribed. He didn't want anything bad to happen to him again.

R_xpert Advice

> ➢ One of the simplest ways to safely lower your drug costs is to use a generic drug. Generic drugs cost much less than the brand-name ones and work the same way. The generic and the brand name are the same drug, but for the generic drug, the patent has expired. For example, Zestril is the brand name for lisinopril and Pravachol is the brand name for pravastatin. Use the generic drug whenever possible.

Many pharmacies now offer generic medications for only $4 for a month's supply. Ask your pharmacist if your drug is available as a generic and if this is right for you.

➤ For problems like high cholesterol, high blood pressure, depression, and stomach pain, lower-cost alternative brand-name drugs are available in place of many high-cost medications. Typically, these drugs are older versions (with the same effect) of newer, more expensive drugs. Some of these drugs may even be available as a generic, saving you even more money! For example, several older statin drugs for high cholesterol like simvastatin and pravastatin have similar effects to the newer brand-name drugs Lipitor and Crestor and may work just as well for you. Ask your doctor if it is appropriate for you to switch to a lower cost alternative drug.

➤ Many drugs that used to be available only by prescription are now available over the counter. These drugs include Prilosec, Prevacid, Zyrtec, Claritin, and others. Ask your doctor and pharmacist if it is okay to take the over-the-counter version of the drug. Your doctor also can tell you if you can switch from the prescription product to one that is similar in an over-the-counter form. For example: Nexium (available only as a prescription) costs approximately $199.99 per month.* An over-the-counter version of a similar drug, Prilosec, costs approximately $22.89 for 42 tablets.* Before you change to an over-the-counter drug, make sure to check with your doctor or pharmacist.

*Retail costs as of 11/2010.

➤ Tablet splitting or "half tabs" may help you save money. Tablet splitting involves buying a higher strength tablet and then splitting it in half to get the correct dose. For example, a 20 mg tablet may cost the same as a 10 mg tablet, so you can save money by buying the 20 mg tablet and cutting it in half. However, if you are easily confused or not able to split tablets safely, this may not be appropriate for you. Ask your pharmacist if you can safely save money by splitting tablets in half.

➤ Most medications contain a single drug; however, some medications contain two or more drugs. Combination drugs can help save you money. For example, if you take hydrochlorothiazide and lisinopril for high blood pressure, you can either buy these as two separate pills or as one combination drug that contains both medications in one pill. The combination drug may be more expensive if you pay out of pocket, but if you have a prescription drug co-pay, you will only have to pay one co-pay for the combination product. This helps to save the cost of one co-pay. Ask your pharmacist if any of your drugs come as a combination product.

➤ Drug Company Patient Assistance Programs (PAP) provide a limited number of brand-name medications to eligible patients at little or no cost. However, there are differences in the way these programs are designed, including the drugs that are covered, a complex application process, income criteria, co-pays, and the length of time you are covered. Check with your pharmacist before signing up for a PAP or go to www. healthassistrx.com for more information about drug company programs.

➤ Several programs offer drug discount cards that can be used for medications that are not covered by insurance, if your co-pay or deductible is high, if the low medication cap has been reached, or if you are in the Medicare Part D donut hole. The cards are not an insurance plan and cannot be used in combination with Medicaid, Medicare, or other state or federal programs that pay for meds. However, you can use the card if you are not using another program to pay for the drug. These cards are only valid at participating pharmacies and may be a good option for high-cost drugs not covered by your insurance plan. Go to www.needymeds.org or www.Rxassist.org for more information regarding drug discount cards.

➤ Buying prescription drugs at a reputable online pharmacy may save you a great deal of money. However, be sure that the pharmacy you use has the VIPPS seal of approval. See safety tip # 31 for more information about buying drugs online.

➤ Herbal products, nutritional supplements, and natural remedies are not cheap. Some of these products sell for $30 or more a bottle. Unfortunately, most of these supplements have not been proven safe *or* effective. Additionally, many supplements and natural products can interact negatively with the prescription drugs you take. Play it safe and ask your doctor or pharmacist if a specific herbal product is safe for you. Otherwise, save your money. These products could be doing you more harm than good.

Bottom Line

There are several ways to lower your drug costs. Using a generic drug, a lower-cost alternative, an over-the-counter med, half tabs, or combination products can help save your money. Still, always ask your pharmacist if these alternatives are safe for you.

Bonus

Go to Reliable Medical Resources in the back of the book for a list of drug company patient-assistance program websites.

Safety Tip #28
Rogue Websites and Cyber Docs: Protect Yourself When Buying Drugs Online

Legitimate websites that sell drugs online can be a convenient, cost-effective way to fill a prescription. Still, you need to be careful to avoid unlicensed online "pharmacies" that sell drugs that may be contaminated, counterfeit, or otherwise unsafe. "Rogue websites" may look like professional and legitimate websites, but they may be covering up for unsafe and illegal pharmacies.

Medicines that come from illegal pharmacies may be

- fake or counterfeit,
- stronger or weaker than they should be,
- expired,
- contaminated with a dangerous product,
- not made properly,
- not labeled properly,
- not stored properly, or
- shipped from countries that do not have safety standards.

Internet pharmacies that ask you to fill out a questionnaire and then have it reviewed by a "cyber doctor" who never sees you may result in a wrong diagnosis and you getting the wrong treatment. The American Medical Association (AMA) and the Food and Drug Administration (FDA) are against this practice because it does not meet accepted standards of medical care. According to the National Association of Boards of Pharmacy (NABP), nearly half of the online pharmacies that use cyber doctors are located outside of the United States, and buying drugs from these pharmacies can be illegal in the United States.

Cyber Doctors

Jerry just wasn't his old self. Recently his sex life had been subpar. He had seen the ads on TV and thought that maybe he had E.D. (erectile dysfunction). But Jerry was too embarrassed to talk to his doctor about it in person. He wasn't comfortable discussing it with anybody.

At work, he overheard a buddy talking about a website where he could get Viagra. He didn't need to talk to a doctor. He just needed to fill out a questionnaire, and the little blue pills would come in the mail. That sounded perfect to Jerry. He got online that night and ordered the Viagra.

A few days later, the pills came in the mail. Jerry took the Viagra and thought his problems were over. Unfortunately, Jerry was running the risk of a severe drug interaction.

Jerry had a history of chest pain, and he took nitroglycerin for his condition. What he didn't know was that nitroglycerin and Viagra would interact with one another and cause his blood pressure to drop dangerously low. Since he had not gotten the prescription for Viagra from his own doctor or had the prescription filled at his pharmacy, he had bypassed all the safety checks that would prevent him from this dangerous interaction.

Buying the Viagra online from the cyber doc bypassed his own doctor knowing that he was taking the drug and his pharmacist from checking for dangerous drug interactions. Buying the Viagra online was a very risky thing for Jerry to do.

R$_x$pert Advice

➤ Do not order medications from an online pharmacy if
  • there is no street address for the pharmacy,
  • there is no phone number for the pharmacy,

- • the pharmacy does not require a prescription, or
- • the prices are much lower than the competition (it sounds too good to be true).

➤ Before you buy your medications online, be sure to check that
  - • the pharmacy is located in the United States,
  - • the state board of pharmacy licenses the Internet pharmacy,
  - • the pharmacy requires a prescription from your doctor,
  - • there is a pharmacist available to answer your questions,
  - • there is a valid phone number for you to call with questions, and
  - • there are valid privacy and security policies in place to protect your health and financial information.

➤ The National Association of Boards of Pharmacy (NABP) identifies pharmacies licensed to sell medicine on the Internet. The program is the Verified Internet Pharmacy Practice Sites or VIPPS. The pharmacy website should display the VIPPS seal of approval. This seal ensures that the pharmacy is a state-licensed pharmacy in good standing and located in the United States. These sites have undergone and successfully completed the NABP accreditation process. This process includes a review of all pharmacy policies and an on-site inspection of the facility. The VIPPS seal also ensures that the online pharmacy meets all state and federal regulations. To check to see if your Internet pharmacy is VIPPS approved, go to www.vipps.info.

➤ Only take medications prescribed for you by the doctor you see in person. Do not take medications prescribed for you by a doctor who does not know you.

➤ Use a licensed online pharmacy displaying the VIPPS seal of approval on their website.

> Be sure the online pharmacy provides a working toll-free phone number so you can call a pharmacist if you have any questions.

> Be sure your credit card and personal health information are private and secure.

> Ask the pharmacist at your local drugstore if he can match or beat the prices of the online pharmacy, then buy it from your local pharmacy.

> Be aware of potential counterfeit medications.

> Check the packaging. If your medicines arrive and the package looks as if it has been opened or changed, do not take them. Call your doctor and get a new prescription.

Bottom Line

Take extra precautions to find a safe online pharmacy to buy your prescription medications. Check to make sure your pharmacy website displays the VIPPS seal of approval. When in doubt, contact the NABP at www.vipps.info to be sure the pharmacy is in good standing.

Safety Tip #29
Little-Known Facts about
Counterfeit Drugs

Counterfeit drugs pose a serious public health risk. The international, multibillion-dollar black market for fake or adulterated drugs is growing at an alarming rate. Innocent patients may unknowingly be taking medicines that do not perform as needed. Some may be fatal.

Some counterfeit drugs actually contain the active ingredients, but many others have the wrong ingredients; little, none, or too much of the active ingredient; or contain dangerous additives. They may carry the brand name or generic label. They may be mislabeled altogether or have fake packaging. Some of these counterfeit products look so much like the actual drug that they fool pharmacists and doctors! No matter how they come, counterfeit drugs are illegal and can result in treatment failure or death.

How Real Is This Problem?

In 2001, a sixteen-year-old boy named Tim Fagan had a liver transplant. At that time, he was prescribed a high-cost injectable drug called Epogen to increase his red blood cells. Following each injection, he experienced severe cramps throughout his entire body. Every time his mother injected a dose, the pain became worse. His doctors did not know what was wrong.

After two months, the family found out that the Epogen that they had been injecting into their son was counterfeit and had been diluted to twenty times below the prescribed dose. The fake packaging on the counterfeit drug was so similar to the real drug that no one, not even the licensed pharmacist down the street who had filled the prescription, could tell them apart.

Mary Sue McAslan, Pharm.D.

This experience was devastating and frightening for Tim and his family and pointed out the severity of taking counterfeit drugs. The Fagan family has gone on to author "Tim Fagan's Law" to combat counterfeit drugs.[16]

R~xpert~ Advice

> You can avoid counterfeit medications by using your common sense. If someone is trying to sell you a drug from a street corner and claiming it's the brand-name drug, assume it's a fraud and walk away.

> Be safe online. If you go to the Internet and find a pharmacy that sells you a prescription drug without a prescription, without a doctor seeing you, and at a very low price, be careful. You may be ordering counterfeit drugs that are not as good as the real drug or may even cause you harm.

> Check to be sure the website you are ordering from displays the VIPPS seal. The VIPPS seal is the benchmark for consumers to ensure the quality of the online pharmacy's practice. Check with www.vipps.info before ordering drugs online.

> If you think that you have a counterfeit drug, do not take it. Take the medication to your pharmacist for verification. Your pharmacist will tell you if there has been a change in manufacturer and if the drug is counterfeit.

> You can report counterfeit drugs to the Food and Drug Administration on their website: www.fda.gov/Safety/MedWatch, or by calling 1-800-332-1088.

Bottom Line

Counterfeit drugs are dangerous and harmful to your health. Don't buy any drug that you think may be counterfeit.

Safety Tip #30
Check, Check, and Double Check: What to Do before You Leave the Pharmacy

The surest way to prevent medication errors at the pharmacy is to open the bag, take out the bottles, open them, and check each bottle before leaving the prescription counter. Check to be sure that your name is on the bottle, that you are getting the right medication in the right quantity, and that you understand the directions. Doing this provides a critical safety check that could possibly save your life.

"I Knew Right Away There Had Been a Mistake"

Kenneth went to the pharmacy to pick up his prescription refills. He asked the pharmacist for his meds and noticed right away that something was wrong. He had ordered several different medications, one being a very large capsule for his cholesterol. He knew that he had ordered ninety pills, and the pharmacist usually had to put them in three large bottles. Normally when he picked up his meds, he had at least two large bags. Today, the pharmacist was handing him a one small prescription bag.

Kenneth opened the bag and took out the pills. "I think there's been a mistake," he said. The pharmacist looked shocked. "I think that you only gave me thirty pills for my cholesterol. I know the prescription is for ninety. Usually, you have to put it into three different bottles."

The pharmacist took back the prescription and sure enough, she had miscounted the pills. Instead of the ninety pills prescribed, she had only given Kenneth thirty. It was a good thing that Kenneth had spoken up. She could correct this situation right away.

Kenneth knew that checking his meds before leaving the counter was the smart thing to do. Today he had caught a big mistake.

Rxpert Advice

➤ When the pharmacist asks if you have any questions, do not say no. Say "Yes, I do" and ask the four NUTS questions. This is especially important for new prescriptions because you are verifying the information that your doctor gave you with the information your pharmacist is giving you. This check helps to prevent you from getting the wrong drug.

➤ Open the prescription bag and make sure the name on the bottle is yours, especially if you have a common last name. This prevents you from getting a drug meant for someone else.

➤ Open the bottle and look at the pills. If they do not look like the ones you have gotten in the past, ask the pharmacist if it is the right drug. The look of a pill (color, shape, markings) may change with different generic manufacturers. It is up to you to be sure that it is the right drug.

➤ Open the bottle and check the number of pills inside. If you were expecting ninety and there are only thirty, then ask the pharmacist why.

➤ Read the directions on the bottle and ask for clarification if you don't understand what they mean. Ask for additional information like what time of day you should take it or if you can take it with food or other meds.

➤ Look at the small brightly colored auxiliary labels. These give you lots of additional information about how to take the medications. These include "Take with Food" and "May Cause Drowsiness."

Bottom Line

Before leaving the prescription counter, stop and open the bag, check the bottles, make sure the pills are for you, in the right quantity, and that you understand exactly how to take them.

Part 4

The Successful Hospital Stay: Preventing Medication Errors in the Hospital

Being a patient in the hospital can be a frightening, confusing, and overwhelming experience. Despite the fact that your doctors and nurses try their best to communicate with you and your advocate, situations may arise where you will need additional help and information to make sure you are getting the care you need. In this section you will learn how to prepare for your hospital stay, how to help coordinate your own care, and how to become the "squeaky wheel" if you need to. This is the key to preventing medication errors in the hospital.

Medication errors are the leading cause of preventable injury in hospitals today. Studies have shown that at least 1.5 million medication errors occur in hospitals each year.[17] On average, that breaks down to at least one medication error per patient in every hospital, every single day.

Don't make the mistake made by most people and blindly hand over control of your care to the hospital staff. You need to be your own advocate, and if you can't, you need to have someone you trust at the ready to speak for you. This section will educate you and the person caring for you on the necessary steps to take to prevent medication errors during your hospital stay.

Safety Tip #31
Not All Hospitals Are Created Equal

You wouldn't buy a used car without kicking the tires first. In fact, you would check its overall performance rating and whether it had been involved in a wreck, and then you would send it to a mechanic for an evaluation. You would do your homework and may even refer to *Consumer Reports* for a detailed automotive comparison and ranking.

Most people spend more time researching a used car than they do a hospital. They choose a hospital because it is close to home or is associated with their health plan, but not all hospitals are created equal.

Take a moment now, before you are hospitalized, to see how your hospital compares to others in your area.

Quality Checkup

Brenda's mom needed heart surgery. Brenda knew her mom would be in the hospital for several days. What Brenda didn't know was which hospital would give her mom the best care.

Brenda asked the doctor for a recommendation. He recommended the large university hospital downtown. He told her that they did many heart surgeries every year and that they had a high quality rating. Brenda wondered why she couldn't take her mom to the small hospital down the street. It would be so much more convenient.

Brenda went online to get more information. She researched both hospitals on www.hospitalcompare.hhs.gov. The large hospital had very high scores for doctor/nurse communication, pain management, explaining medications, and patient satisfaction. The small hospital had considerably lower scores in all categories.

Brenda then went to www.healthgrades.com where she was able to check how the smaller hospital compared to the larger hospital in success rates for heart surgeries. The large hospital had five stars, the best possible ranking, and the smaller hospital had only one star, the lowest possible ranking. When Brenda took her mom to the university hospital, she felt good about her doctor's recommendation and confident that her mom would be getting the best care possible.

R𝗑pert Advice

> If you have more than one hospital or surgical center to choose from, ask your doctor which one he or she prefers, and which one would be the best for you. This is especially important if you are having a complex surgery or other invasive treatment.

> Ask your doctor or contact the hospital yourself and ask how often the hospital does the type of surgery that you need. If they do not perform that procedure very often, find another hospital that does. For example, if you need complicated heart surgery, find the surgeon and the hospital that performs most of these surgeries in your area every year.

> Ask the doctor or hospital representative about the hospital's experience in taking care of people with your illness. You would want them to have taken care of many people with the same condition as you.

> Ask what special type of care the hospital provides for people with your type of illness. Are they set up to give you additional care that you may need?

Bottom Line

Perform a quality checkup on each of your hospital choices before you decide where to go. When you ask these questions, you can help make sure that you or someone you care for has the best treatment possible.

Bonus

Go to www.drmarysue.com for additional websites to help you perform a quality check on your hospital.

Safety Tip #32
Two Heads Are Better than One: Line Up an Advocate

If you're a patient in a hospital, your main job is to get well. Having an advocate, (spouse, child, or trusted friend) to watch over you and help with some of the difficult details, is vital to your care and the prevention of errors before, during, and after your hospital stay.

An advocate is someone that you designate to speak for you with your doctors, nurses, and other health-care providers. Your advocate can ask questions, interpret the answers, take notes, help you communicate your wishes, and then remember and understand confusing and sometimes fearful information. Your advocate may be your caregiver (that person who helps take care of you on a daily basis), it may be a third party, or it may be a child or concerned friend. Either way, this person has agreed to step up and advocate for you. It is up to your advocate to act on your behalf and to speak up and get the answers you need. It is their responsibility to keep you well informed and safe.

Rest Easy

Helen was the caregiver and advocate for her eighty-five-year-old mother, Sophia. Helen kept track of her mother's medical records, including her health history, current problems, insurance information, and medications. She also helped coordinate her mother's care between her primary care doctor and several different specialists.

Sophia was scheduled for hip replacement surgery the next week. Helen knew that as her mother's advocate, she needed to prepare for this. She read up on the surgery so that she knew what to expect and jotted down several questions to ask the doctor before the hospital admission. She made sure that the insurance coverage was up-to-date and that she had the necessary documentation to take with her. Helen also reviewed all of her mom's medications and made certain that the med list included her prescription and over-the-counter drugs. She put everything in the Personal Health System binder so that she would have everything in one place and ready to go.

Helen and Sophia checked into the hospital. After the surgery, Helen took it upon herself to stay at her mother's bedside to make sure things ran smoothly. She was there to ask questions when the nurses brought in new medications, and Helen made sure she knew what the medications were for and what to expect from them. She was also there to request pain meds when her mother was unable to. She was there to speak with the different doctors and nurses regarding her mother's treatment. Because Helen was there to advocate for her mother, Sophia had a successful hospital stay.

Before leaving the hospital, Helen was told that her mother would require an injection of a blood thinner for several days after she got home. Helen would have to inject the medication into the skin on her mother's abdomen. Helen had never given a shot before and this made her very uneasy, but if she didn't do this, who would? Helen was trained by the nurses to give the injection, and after practicing a few times she felt confident that she could do this. Helen was also told that she would have to watch her mother for any bruising or bleeding and call the doctor if there were any problems.

Sophia did not know what she would have done without Helen. As her advocate, she had allowed Sophia to rest easy, and ensured that everything had gone smoothly before, during, and after her surgery.

R̶xpert Advice

Your advocate plays a vital role before, during, and after your hospital stay.

Before your hospital admission, your advocate can do the following:

➢ Call the insurance company before your hospital stay. The phone number of the insurance company is on the back of the insurance ID card, but you can make it easy to find if you include this number on the Emergency Health Profile.

➢ Keep a copy of your Personal Health System and help you fill out an updated medication list. It should include all of the prescription medicines and over-the-counter medications that you take. Include any herbal products and vitamins or natural supplements, as well as any drugs that you buy at the drugstore, grocery store, health food store, and nutritional products stores. In addition to the medications you take, the med list should include any medications you are allergic to, including tape and latex. It is very important that you bring this information with you to the hospital. The Personal Health System also lists past medications, tests, and other information that is vital to your care.

➢ Update and keep a copy of your Emergency Health Profile. Once filled out, this form has all of your insurance information and the insurance company's customer service number. In an emergency, your advocate should contact your insurance company as soon as possible to confirm coverage.

➢ Your advocate can research your medications and illness. This may include online websites, the library, or support groups.

➢ Ask your doctor about the special training and experience that he has received in treating your illness.

➢ Seek and obtain a second opinion if needed. Never be afraid to get a second opinion. These are standard practice and can lead to a more appropriate treatment plan.

➢ Read medical consent forms and make sure that you understand them before signing anything. If you or your advocate does not understand the medical forms, get the doctor or nurse to explain them to you.

➢ Know and advocate for your wishes. While circumstances may cause a change of plan, your advocate should be able to weigh the relevance of any new information and its impact on your wishes for your care.

➢ Communicate with your health-care proxy. This is the person you designate to make decisions about your care if you are unable to make them on your own.

During your hospital stay, your advocate can do the following:

➢ Stay with you. You will feel reassured having your advocate stay with you as long as possible while you are hospitalized, even overnight. If you are unable to make your wishes or needs known, your advocate can speak for you and let you rest.

➢ Make sure you get the right medications and treatments. Be sure your advocate is present when you are receiving medications so they can monitor whether the medication is working or not and if you are having side effects.

➢ Ask questions that you will not think of or remember to ask when you are ill. Your advocate also will remember the answers and be able to write them down along with any additional information that is discussed. This will be important information to have if there are any questions after you get home.

➢ Communicate with your health-care providers on your behalf. Choose a person who will cooperate with the medical staff for your best care. It is very important that this person understands the type of care and treatments that you want and will respect your decisions.

After your hospital stay, your advocate can do the following:

➢ Know what care you will need once you get home. Have your advocate ask about your follow-up appointments and, when possible, make these appointments before you leave the hospital.

➢ Be sure that you understand all instructions regarding medications and know what to do (and who to call) if there is a problem or if you have a side effect or an allergic reaction to a medication. If you will be using oxygen or any other medical equipment, your advocate can be sure that you know how to use this equipment and who to call if you don't understand.

Bottom Line

It is up to your advocate to speak up on your behalf to be sure that you receive the correct care and treatment you need.

Safety Tip #33
Coordinate Your Care: What Your Doctor Wants You to Do

One of the biggest causes of medication errors in our hospitals is the lack of communication and coordination between all of the staff that take care of you during your hospital stay.[18] Many times it's a problem of "one hand not knowing what the other hand is doing," leading to serious gaps and mistakes. There are certain things that your doctor wants you to do to help prevent these mistakes from happening during your hospital stay.

"*Stop*—I Think There's Been a Mistake"

Joe's hospital stay had gone well so far. He had been admitted for a severe headache the day before, and the treatment was working well. He was resting comfortably.

The doctor came in and told Joe that he wanted to order one more test just to be sure everything was okay—an MRI, which was a scan of the brain. The doctor told Joe that he would be given a "contrast agent" that they would inject intravenously to help see the images of his brain more clearly.

Something did not seem right. Joe remembered that several years ago he had been given something during an X-ray that had caused a severe allergic reaction. He had almost stopped breathing.

Joe spoke up and told his doctor about it. He asked his doctor if he would be given the same agent and whether it would cause another allergic reaction. The doctor immediately noted the allergy in Joe's chart and specifically ordered the MRI to be done without the contrast agent. The doctor was glad that Joe had told him about the allergy. Joe felt relieved.

Joe was taken to the radiology department for the MRI. The radiology technician began to explain the MRI procedure and told Joe that first, he would be given an IV contrast agent to help enhance the images. Joe was shocked! He told the technician to *stop* and call the doctor. There had been a mistake. He was allergic to the contrast agent, and he was sure the doctor had ordered the MRI to be done without it.

The technician was accustomed to giving a contrast agent when doing an MRI, so he hadn't checked Joe's chart. When he went back to the chart for a closer look, there it was. Joe was right. The doctor had specifically ordered the MRI without the contrast agent. In this case, two opportunities for a serious medical mistake were averted because Joe was willing to speak up and provide his doctor and the radiology technician with information that was critical to his health.

R$_x$pert Advice

> Lack of coordination of your care between multiple doctors leads to confusion and miscommunication. Your doctor wants you to designate one primary doctor who will coordinate all of your care. This will help prevent multiple and unnecessary tests and medications. If you need more help, ask to speak to the case manager, patient advocate, or social worker. They should help with coordinating your care.

> Medication mistakes are the biggest cause of injury for hospital patients. This is especially true when you are being moved from one area of the hospital to another. Your doctor wants you to be aware of mistakes if you are being moved to a different floor or unit.

> If you do not understand why you are being given a drug or treatment, test or procedure, your doctor wants you to stop and ask *why*. Do not stop asking *why* until you have the answers that you and your advocate need to completely understand your treatment. If the nurse cannot answer your

questions, then ask for the nursing supervisor. If she cannot answer your questions, then ask to speak to your doctor. You have the right to get the answers you need.

➤ Your doctor wants you to know why you are in the hospital and what your treatment plan is.

➤ Your doctor wants you or your advocate to keep track of tests and treatments, especially at night and on weekends when there may be fewer staff on duty.

➤ Your doctor wants you to know that "if it doesn't seem right to you, it probably isn't." *Stop* and ask *what* and *why* something is happening. Unless it is a critical, emergency situation, generally you will have the time to get the answers you need.

Bottom Line

Your doctor wants you to ask questions and keep track of your treatments, medications, and tests. This will help coordinate your care among all of your health-care providers and decrease the possibility of medication and other hospital-related errors. You or your advocate must provide the last safety check in your overall treatment and care.

Safety Tip #34
A Checklist for a Safe Hospital Stay

If you are scheduled for a hospital admission, it is up to you or your advocate to take time to prepare. Serious medication errors have occurred because the patient did not know what to do or did not prepare adequately for the hospital stay. Knowing what to do, including updating your medication list and other health records, is critical to preventing errors as well as contributing to a safe and comfortable hospital stay.

Jenny Was Ready

Jenny was having surgery tomorrow. The nurse in her doctor's office had given her written instructions regarding what she could eat and drink, what medications she should and should not take before she came to the hospital, and what time to arrive. Jenny had updated her medication list and the information in her Personal Health System. She had packed some comfortable clothes, leaving any valuable jewelry or personal items at home. She was prepared and ready to go.

The next morning, Jenny got up and took all of her medications like she always did, including her blood thinner. When she arrived at the hospital, the doctor asked her if she had taken her medications that morning. Jenny replied that she had. The doctor was concerned because he knew the blood thinner could cause serious bleeding during the surgery. He also knew that there were specific directions about medications on the information sheet that his nurse had given to Jenny, but somehow she had not understood this.

The doctor decided that it was not safe to perform the surgery that day and canceled the procedure. Despite the fact that Jenny had taken the time to prepare for her hospital stay, she had misunderstood one important piece of information, causing her to reschedule for another day.

R_xpert Advice

> One of the most important things to do prior to a hospital admission is to ask your doctor what medications you should or should not take before you get there. This includes prescription medications, vitamins, over-the-counter drugs, herbal products, nutritional supplements, natural remedies, and all other meds you take.

> It is important that you update your medication list before your surgery and that you notify your doctor of any medication allergies, especially new allergies that he may not be aware of.

> Ask your doctor if there are any foods or beverages (including alcohol) that you need to avoid before your procedure.

> It is best to keep all of your important medical information on hand for your doctor to review during your hospital stay. The Personal Health System will help you and your caregiver or advocate keep track of all of this information.

Use this checklist to be sure you bring everything you will need (and leave home what you won't need).

What to Bring

✓ medical documents—including advanced directives, durable power of attorney, and living will

✓ test results—including lab tests, X-rays, and other information your doctor wants you to bring

✓ insurance card or health plan card

✓ identification (You may need your driver's license for identification upon admission. However, have your caregiver keep this for you during your stay.)

✓ updated list of all of your medications (including prescription drugs, over-the-counter drugs, vitamins, herbals remedies, and nutritional supplements) and a complete list of all your medication allergies

✓ list of phone numbers of family members, designated medical advocate, and close friends

✓ list of your regular doctors by name, including phone numbers

✓ notepad and pen to write down questions for your doctor and nurses

✓ small amount of money ($10) for magazines and other small purchases

✓ eyeglasses or contact lenses (Remember to bring contact lens solutions if needed.)

✓ reading materials—books, magazines, crossword puzzles, etc.

✓ bathrobe and slippers, loose-fitting pajamas or nightgown, short-sleeved bed jacket or cardigan sweater, underwear, and socks

✓ toiletries—deodorant, lip balm, toothpaste and toothbrush, lotion, shampoo, soap, comb, and brush

What *not* to Bring Leave It at Home!

Leave your credit cards, cash, and jewelry at home. You won't be doing much shopping or attending many galas during your hospital stay.

Check before You Bring

Before you bring in electronic devices, check your hospital's policy. Generally, cell phones are not allowed because they interfere with hospital monitors. Get permission from your nurse before you use laptop computers, DVD players, and electronic reading devices. These may be allowed, yet they are also targets for theft. If you want to bring them, make sure you can safely secure these devices while you are sleeping or not in your room.

Bottom Line

Before you check in, check list. Be prepared. Follow the checklist to ensure a safe and comfortable hospital stay.

Safety Tip # 35
Your Emergency Health Profile:
Don't Leave Home without It!

In the event of an emergency, the Emergency Health Profile can help save your life. This form contains your vital health information all in one place. See the back of the book for a copy of the Emergency Health Profile or download a copy on www.drmarysue.com. Be sure it is filled out before an emergency arises so the information is accurate, complete, and readily available. Keep this form with you and give a copy to your caregivers and emergency contacts. In an emergency, this form can be a lifesaver.

The Emergency Health Profile includes the following:

- ✓ your name, address, phone numbers, date of birth, primary language spoken
- ✓ emergency contact information
- ✓ medical problems
- ✓ medication list and medication allergies
- ✓ doctors' information
- ✓ insurance information

"Are You Allergic to Any Pain Meds?"

Susan did not feel well. She had a high fever and a horrible headache. Susan called her doctor who told her to go to the emergency room for treatment. Since Susan felt so badly, she did not have time to gather her insurance information or other important medical documents. She was in no condition to sit down and make a list of her medications.

Susan's husband, Ryan, kept a copy of Susan's Emergency Health Profile. It listed her medications, allergies, and her insurance information. He made sure he had it before he took Susan to the hospital.

At the emergency room, the admissions clerk asked Susan for her insurance card. She also asked what medications Susan was taking and if she had any allergies. Susan felt so awful she could not remember any of this information. She just needed something for the pain.

Ryan was able to give the admissions clerk the Emergency Health Profile. It listed all of the information the clerk was asking for. She was glad Ryan had it, as it would make Susan's admission process much quicker and easier.

The emergency room doctor examined Susan and wanted to give her something for pain right away. The doctor asked Susan if she had any allergies to pain meds but Susan could not remember. Ryan showed the doctor the Emergency Health Profile because he knew it listed her allergies, including codeine.

The doctor was glad that Ryan had the form. It listed the codeine allergy and all of the other medications Susan was taking. By reviewing the list, he could safely administer a pain med that Susan was not allergic to and would not interact with the other meds she was taking. The doctor wished everyone came to the ED so prepared.

R$_x$pert Advice

➢ Trying to complete complicated medical forms and answer confusing medical questions during a time of stress is very difficult and may lead to wrong or incomplete information and medical errors. Fill out the Emergency Health Profile before you really need it.

➢ Make arrangements beforehand to be sure it gets into the hands of emergency medical techs (EMTs) and emergency room personnel. Keep one in your glove compartment, purse, or briefcase. Be sure your caregivers and emergency contacts have a copy of this form before an emergency occurs.

> ➤ Make sure you have an Emergency Health Profile ready for each of your loved ones. Keep your own copies of this form for your spouse, parents, children, and others. You never know when you will need it.

Bonus

Go to www.drmarysue.com to download a copy of the Emergency Health Profile.

Safety Tip #36
Be the Squeaky Wheel:
Ask Questions and Get the
Answers You Need

It's easy to be intimidated by doctors, nurses, and other hospital staff, but when your health or the health of someone you care for is the issue, this is not the time to back down. If you have any questions or concerns about any aspect of your health-care treatment, *stop*, ask questions, and get the answers you need before going any further with any medications or treatments.

Just Say No!

Nancy was recuperating in her hospital bed at 7:30 a.m. the day after her surgery. She was in pain, and the night-shift nurse had just given her a pain pill. She was starting to feel a little better now.

The day-shift nurse came into her room at 8:30 a.m. and told Nancy it was time for her pain pill. Nancy told the nurse that the night-shift nurse had given her the pain pill an hour ago. She did not need another one.

The day-shift nurse insisted that the pain pill had not been given since it was not written down on her chart. It was her job to give it, and Nancy had to take it. Nancy again said she did not need it or want it because she had been given one already. The nurse would not take "no" for an answer and insisted that Nancy take the potent pain medication. Nancy felt intimidated by the nurse. Although she knew this was not right, Nancy gave in to the pressure and just took the pill.

A short while later, Nancy felt lightheaded, nauseated, sleepy, and dizzy. She called for the head nurse. Nancy told her that the day shift nurse had refused to listen to her when she tried to tell her she did not need a second pain pill. As a result, Nancy had gotten an overdose and was feeling worse than before.

Nancy learned the hard way not to give in to pressure. She knew that she would need to stick up for herself if something didn't seem right. If that didn't work, she would ask to speak to the head nurse or her doctor.

R$_x$pert Advice

> ➢ Make sure that you and your advocate completely understand why you are being given the medication, what you can expect from it, and when you should start to see results.
> ➢ Ask your doctor or nurse for the name of the new medication.
> ➢ Ask your doctor or nurse why you are being given this medication.
> ➢ Ask your doctor or nurse about the side effects of the medication.
> ➢ Ask your doctor or nurse when you should start feeling better.
> ➢ Ask your doctor or nurse to provide any written information about the new drug.
> ➢ Ask your doctor or nurse if the hospital provides patient education.
> ➢ Tell your doctor if you have ever had an allergic reaction to any medications (rash, swelling, shortness of breath, etc.).
> ➢ Tell your doctor if you have had any side effects or reactions to any medications (nausea, dizziness, etc.).
> ➢ Ask questions until you completely understand why you are getting a certain medication or treatment. Don't back down. If you don't get the answers you need, ask to speak to the supervisor or your doctor.

➤ Pay attention to your care and make sure you are getting the right medication or treatment at the right time by the right staff. If you cannot do this for yourself, ask your advocate for help.

➤ Keep a journal or log of your medications and treatments, highlighting any issues you want to be sure are not overlooked by the staff. This may include changes in medications, new allergic reactions or side effects, and information that your doctor or nurse tells you about your plan of care.

➤ Know who will be taking care of you.

➤ Know how long the treatment should last and how you should feel. Understand that more tests or more medications may not be the solution for you. Ask your doctor if these are really necessary.

➤ Never be afraid to ask for a second opinion. In most cases, you will have time to get a second opinion. The more information you have, the more secure you will feel about the decisions you make.

Bottom Line:

Be the squeaky wheel. Don't be afraid to speak up and ask questions. Demand that you get the answers you need. Don't stop asking until you completely understand why a treatment or medication is being given.

Safety Tip #37
Can You Please Repeat That?

If you don't understand medical jargon or the complicated terms and abbreviations used by medical professionals, speak up and let them know you don't understand. Never nod your head and pretend you understand. Many people don't have a clue what their doctor is telling them, even when the doctor is giving them vital information about their medications, treatments, procedures, illness, or disease.

Medical information is very complicated, and understanding it requires knowledge that most people don't have. Many patients do not understand what is being discussed during the informed consent process or the issues surrounding a second opinion. When this information comes up, patients often are nervous, anxious, scared, worried, and can't concentrate. To make matters worse, add to that a language barrier, and almost all of the medical information can get lost in translation. Unfortunately, this lack of understanding of medical information can result in catastrophic outcomes.

He Didn't Understand a Word She Said

After a week in the hospital, Luis was ready to go home. The nurse told him that the pharmacist would be in to see him and review his medications before he left. Luis hoped the pharmacist would hurry up. He wanted to go.

The pharmacist came in to see Luis with a new list of the medications he would be taking once he got home. She wanted to make sure Luis would take his new medications correctly, so one by one, she reviewed each medication, telling him the name of the drug, what it was for, how to take it, and which side effects were dangerous. Unfortunately, Luis never learned to read or understand English very well. Spanish was his first language. In fact, Luis did not understand one word the pharmacist was saying. She used too many big words and they all sounded very confusing.

When the pharmacist asked Luis if he understood, he simply nodded his head "yes." The pharmacist wasn't fooled; she knew Luis did not understand. Luis's doctor was relying on her to communicate this important medical information to him so that he would avoid another hospital admission.

The pharmacist told Luis that she would be right back and left the room. When she returned, she brought a Spanish-speaking pharmacist who helped to translate some of the more complicated information. She handed Luis written instructions printed in Spanish. Luis could read and understand these materials. They even had pictures and charts that would help Luis to take his medications at the right time. The pharmacist asked Luis to repeat back the instructions so she could be certain he understood them. Luis was able to do this without any problems.

Luis left the hospital armed with written information in his own language that would help him to take his medications correctly. Everyone—the doctor, the pharmacist, and especially Luis—felt confident that he would take his medications correctly and avoid another trip to the hospital.

℞pert Advice

- If you have trouble understanding what your doctors and other health-care providers are telling you, it is up to you to say "Stop!" and let them know that you do not understand. Don't be embarrassed or worried. Just ask them to repeat the information or say it another way that you can understand.
- Try to be specific as to what you don't understand. Keep asking until the information is clear.
- Your caregiver plays a very important role. Ask your caregiver to write down all of the information.

➤ Ask for written drug or treatment information in your native language or an easy-to-read format, for you to take home.

➤ Tell the nurse or pharmacist if you do not know how or when to take your medications. If a family member or friend helps you take your medicine, be sure to have the nurse or pharmacist speak with your caregiver about your medications.

➤ If you speak another language, ask for someone who speaks your language. You have the right to get free help from someone who speaks your language.

➤ If you have trouble reading, do not be embarrassed. Speak up and ask for easy-to-read materials or have the information read to you.

Bottom Line

Do not leave the hospital until you completely understand the medical information your doctor, pharmacist, nurse, and other health-care providers have given you.

Safety Tip #38
There's Only One You:
Prevent Patient Mix-ups

One of the most common and most dangerous medication errors in the hospital is a patient mix-up, which is when one patient is confused with another patient and receives a medication by mistake. Two patients may have the same last name, physically look alike, or simply be in the same room and receive a drug not meant for them.

Accurate patient identification is especially important if you have a common last name. When two or more patients on the same hospital floor have the same last name, the odds of error go way up. Stop and tell the nurse if you think she has you confused with another patient with the same last name.

Below is a list of the top ten most common last names in the United States.* If your name is on this list, you are at a higher risk of patient mix-up.

1) Smith	6) Miller
2) Johnson	7) Davis
3) Williams	8) Garcia
4) Brown	9) Rodriguez
5) Jones	10) Wilson

*www.census.gov (November 2010)

"Good Morning, Mr. Johnson"

John Johnson was on wing 3 east in room 315, bed B. Tom Johnson was also on 3 east and was in room 320, bed A. The nurse on duty, Linda, began to hand out the morning medications. She entered John Johnson's room and introduced herself. She said, "Good morning, Mr. Johnson" and checked his wristband to be sure she had the right patient. Sure enough, his wristband said "Johnson." Linda gave John Johnson three pills and a shot of insulin. She left the room and proceeded with giving medications to the rest of the patients on her floor.

A few moments later, she entered Tom Johnson's room. *Hmm,* she thought. She hadn't noticed that she had two Mr. Johnsons on her floor. She had not verified the full name of Mr. Johnson in room 315. She had only checked his wristband to be sure it said "Johnson." She became alarmed when she realized that she had just given the wrong medication, including a shot of insulin, to John Johnson.

Linda immediately contacted the nursing supervisor and the doctor and told them about the error. The doctor told her that the insulin shot would cause John Johnson's blood sugar to drop rapidly and gave her instructions for monitoring and treating low blood sugar. Due to this medication error, John Johnson could be in serious danger.

John Johnson recovered completely from this error, but later said that he knew something just didn't seem right. The medications he had been given didn't look familiar to him, and he had not known why he was getting a shot of insulin. He told his doctor that he should have spoken up and asked what the meds were and why he was getting them. He should have made sure that the nurse checked his wristband and that she had the right patient. John Johnson learned to speak up and make sure the nurse and the rest of the staff had the right "Mr. Johnson" from now on. He didn't want any more mistakes happening to him or the other Mr. Johnson.

Mary Sue McAslan, Pharm.D.

R_xpert Advice

> Expect your doctor, nurse, and all other health-care providers to introduce themselves to you. If they do not introduce themselves, ask them who they are.

> Expect that your doctor, nurse, and all other health-care providers will check your wristband and another form of identification to verify who you are before giving you any medications or doing any blood tests or procedures.

> Hospitals use two different methods for patient identification. This may include your full name and full social security number, your date of birth, or your address. Be sure the nurse and other health-care personnel verify your identity in two ways before you accept any medications or treatments.

> Be patient when a doctor, nurse, pharmacist, lab technician, X-ray technician, and all other hospital staff ask you to repeat your full name and other identifiers. This may seem tedious for you, but they are doing their job making sure that you are the right patient getting the right tests, treatments, or drugs.

> Don't hesitate to tell the nurse if you think she has confused you with another patient, and you think you are about to get the wrong medicine.

Bottom Line

Pay attention to the care you are receiving in the hospital and speak up if you think the nurse or other health-care providers have confused you with another patient.

Safety Tip #39
Keep Tabs on Your Meds

Medication errors in the hospital occur frequently when checking in or out of the hospital or being moved from one unit or floor to another. These errors include getting a drug meant for someone else, getting the wrong drug or the wrong dose, getting the drug at the wrong time, or not getting the drug at all. While you are in the hospital, you or your advocate should know which medications you should be getting, why you are getting them, and when you should get them.

Infusion Confusion

Debbie was the caregiver and advocate for her grandmother, Edna Jones. Edna had a fever and was having difficulty breathing. Her doctor told her to go to the emergency room immediately.

Debbie was prepared. Her grandmother took thirteen different prescription medications, including eye drops, inhalers, and creams. She also took an over-the-counter antacid, laxative, pain reliever, calcium supplement, multivitamin, vitamin D, Saint-John's-wort, and fish oil. Debbie had all of these listed on her grandmother's medication list. She also listed her grandmother's medication allergies on the form, which included penicillin.

Debbie checked in at the emergency room admissions desk. A few minutes later, her grandmother was taken back to be examined. Debbie accompanied her grandmother, who was not feeling well enough to answer the doctor's questions.

The ER doctor examined Edna and asked what medications she was currently taking. Debbie showed the doctor the med list. The doctor decided to admit Edna to the hospital so that she could receive IV antibiotics to fight off the chest infection.

Edna was admitted to the fourth-floor nursing unit. The doctor prescribed an IV antibiotic for Edna. Debbie asked the nurse if the IV antibiotic was penicillin. She told the nurse that her grandmother was allergic to penicillin. The nurse checked the order and was surprised to see that the prescribed antibiotic was a form of penicillin. The ER doctor had not documented the allergy in the chart, and the doctor on the unit had prescribed it for her. The nurse contacted the doctor, who changed the order to a different antibiotic.

Later that evening, Edna was sleeping when the nurse came in with the IV. The nurse was in the process of hanging the IV when she gently nudged Edna and said, "Miss Smith, I'm here to hang your IV."

Debbie sat up and said, "This is Edna Jones, not Miss Smith. Who is Miss Smith?" From the next bed, a faint voice said, "I'm Nancy Smith." Debbie was stunned. The nurse was about to give her grandmother an IV meant for the woman in the next bed. The nurse had not even looked at her grandmother's wristband and did not even try to verify her grandmother's name.

A half hour later, another nurse came into the room with the correct IV. The nurse identified herself and told Debbie that she was there to start the IV antibiotic for her grandmother, Edna Jones. The nurse verified Edna's name on her wristband and asked Edna to repeat her full name. The nurse proceeded to hang the IV and told Debbie that it would take approximately one hour for the IV to run in. It was critical that her grandmother get this medication to fight off the infection.

An hour later when Debbie checked the IV bag, she was perplexed. The bag was still full. In fact, there did not seem to be any liquid running in the IV tubing. Debbie called the nurse, who then came to check the IV. To the nurse's dismay, she realized she had not remembered to unclamp the tubing that connected the bag to Edna's arm. Edna had not received any of the medication.

Debbie was extremely frustrated and angry. Her grandmother had been in the hospital for only a few hours and she already had been prescribed a drug she was allergic to, almost received a medication for her roommate, and now the tubing to receive the correct medication hadn't even been unclamped! What more could go wrong? She hoped her grandmother survived her hospital stay.

R_xpert Advice

> When being given drugs in the hospital, ask the doctor or nurse what they are and what they are supposed to treat. Do not take a drug without being told the reason for the drug.

> Ask your caregiver to be present whenever you are receiving medications. This is especially important if you are unable to check for yourself.

> Ask about the side effects of the medication and what you should do if you think you are having a side effect.

> If you do not recognize a medication that is being given to you, ask the nurse to double-check that the medication is for you *before* you take the drug. Never take a drug and then ask if it is correct.

> Read the label on the IV bag. Make sure the IV has your name on it. If you cannot read the label, ask your caregiver to read it for you.

> Ask your nurse how long it should take the IV to run out. If it does not seem to be running, call the nurse right away and let her know.

> Keep a log or journal of the drugs you are being given. This will help prevent confusion, especially if you are transferred from one unit or floor to another.

> Ask to speak to a pharmacist about your medications. Pharmacists can help to decrease medication errors, spot potentially harmful drug interactions, and alert you to dangerous side effects.

Bottom Line

Medication errors and near misses can happen at any time during your hospital stay. Keep track of which drugs you are taking. Know when you should be taking your medications and the proper doses, and always know why you are taking a drug before you take it.

Safety Tip # 40
Critical Communication:
Questions to Ask Your Nurse

Staff nurses are some of the busiest people in the hospital. They may be responsible for handing out hundreds of medications to dozens of patients each day. It's no wonder that medication errors can happen so easily. Mistakes can include getting a drug meant for someone else, getting a drug at the wrong time, getting the wrong dose, or not getting the drug at all.

Oops! Wrong Room!

My father suffered from dementia and was admitted to the hospital for pneumonia. My mom was his caregiver and advocate. Mom was at the bedside when one of the nurses came in with a medicine cup containing five pills.

"I'm here to give Mr. Smith his medication."

"What medication is that?" my mom asked, knowing Dad usually did not take any medications at that time of day.

"I'm not really sure," she said, "but I have to give them."

My mom stood her ground. "This doesn't seem right. Would you mind double-checking the medication orders before you give them?"

The nurse stomped out of the room. She returned a few minutes later and snatched back the medication cup. "Oops!" she said. "Wrong room." She spun on her heels and whizzed out of my dad's room.

My mom had just stopped the nurse from administering five medications meant for someone else to my dad who was critically ill. Had she not spoken up, a medical mistake would have occurred to possibly a tragic outcome.

R${}_x$pert Advice

➢ Know your nurse by name and make sure she knows yours. If there is any doubt that you are not the right patient, or that you are not getting the right drug, at the right time, or at the right dose, tell your nurse that you will not take the drug until she has confirmed that this med is for you.

➢ If something does not seem right and your nurse cannot answer your questions to your satisfaction, *stop* and demand that your concerns be addressed by someone who can.

➢ Verify that you are the correct patient before taking any medication. Hospitals should use two different ways to identify you. Make sure the nurse checks your wristband and verifies your full name each time she gives you a medication.

➢ Ask your nurse the name of the drug. If you do not recognize the drug, ask the nurse to double-check that the drug is for you. Simply say, "That drug does not look familiar to me. Would you mind checking to be sure it is for me?"

➢ Ask your nurse why you are getting the drug. Make sure that the information makes sense and matches what your doctor told you.

➢ Ask your nurse when you will be getting the drug. Is the drug scheduled for a certain time every day or given only when needed? Know the time the medication should be given and if you don't get it on time, tell your nurse.

➢ Doses often are missed when patients leave the floor for tests. If you believe you have missed a dose of your medications, or if there has been a delay, speak up. Most of the time, it is important that you receive your drugs at a specific time. If your doctor told you that you will be getting a medication and you do not get it, ask your nurse to check it. The order for your medication may have been lost or delayed.

➤ Tell your nurse if you are about to get too much. Ask her to check the order to be sure you get the right dose.

➤ Ask your nurse to explain the drug's possible side effects and what to do if you have one. If you think you are having a side effect, tell your nurse. She should contact the doctor, and you may get a different medication.

➤ Ask for help immediately if you think you are having a side effect or an allergic reaction.

➤ Before the nurse gives you any medication, tell her if you have medication allergies or if you have had a bad reaction to a drug. This is especially important if this is a new allergy or reaction as the information may not have been communicated between the nursing staff.

➤ Ask your nurse when you should start to feel better and what you should do if you do not feel better.

➤ Ask your nurse for any written information about the drug.

➤ If you are being given an IV medication, ask your nurse how long it should take the IV to run in. A large IV bag may take several hours, while a small bag may take only thirty to sixty minutes. Tell the nurse if it looks like it's not dripping.

➤ Insist that anyone who touches you—medical staff, nursing staff, visitors, and family—has washed his or her hands. You will see dispensers of antibacterial hand sanitizer on the wall. If you don't see them use it, ask if they have.

Bottom Line

If anything about your medication seems wrong to you, tell your nurse that you will not take it until she has made sure it is right. This includes the right drug, the right dose, the right time, and that you are the right patient.

Safety Tip # 41
Shift Change—A Highly Error-Prone Time of Day

Shift change—when one shift of nurses is going off duty and another shift of nurses is coming on—is one of the most highly error-prone times of day in the hospital. Nurses are extremely busy during this time of day as they try to coordinate and communicate the details of care for an entire floor of patients to the next shift of nurses coming on duty. Dangerous medication errors and oversights often occur during this time.

Shift Change—Time to Speak Up

It was 7:00 a.m. and Tom was just waking up in his hospital room. Tom's night-shift nurse came in to give him his morning dose of insulin. She gave him the insulin and told Tom that she was going home for the day and would see him later that night.

About thirty minutes later, the day-shift nurse came in and prepared to give Tom another dose of his morning insulin.

"Why are you giving me another dose of insulin?" Tom asked.

"I'm giving you your morning dose," she said.

"The night nurse just gave it to me," Tom replied. Tom knew that his blood sugar would drop dangerously low if he had two shots of insulin in less than one hour.

The day-shift nurse stopped and checked Tom's chart. The night-shift nurse had failed to sign off on the morning dose. There was no mention of Tom receiving his insulin in the medication chart. Additionally, during the busy shift change, the night nurse had forgotten to tell anyone that she had already given Tom his insulin.

Because Tom knew what time he was supposed to get his insulin and what changes it caused in his body, he knew he would have become very ill if he had received a second dose. There had been a lack of communication between the two nursing shifts, and by speaking up, Tom had stopped a dangerous error from happening to him.

R_xpert Advice

> ➢ Find out the shift-change times on your unit or floor. You will know it's a shift change when one shift of nurses goes home and a new shift of nurses comes on duty.

> ➢ Learn the names of the nurses who are leaving and of those nurses coming on duty.

> ➢ Pay attention to the medications you are supposed to get, especially during or near a shift change. If you are expecting to receive a medication and do not get it, ask your nurse when you will get it. It may have been overlooked.

> ➢ If you are unable to monitor when you are supposed to get your medications, ask your advocate to help keep track and make sure you are getting the right medication at the right time.

> ➢ Be sure either you or your advocate can communicate critical information that needs to be shared from one shift of nurses to the next, like new allergies or bad reactions to a drug.

Bottom Line

Shift change is an extremely error-prone time of day in the hospital. Be sure that critical information is communicated from one shift of nurses and doctors to the next.

Safety Tip #42
What to Do before Filing a Complaint

What should you do if there's been a mistake and you want someone know about it? There are two options for filing a complaint:

1) File the complaint internally within the hospital.

2) File the complaint externally with an outside organization.

If you need to file a complaint, you are more likely to get the results you want if you follow certain procedures. Following the story are the steps you should apply to filing a complaint against a hospital for quality-of-care issues, which include medication errors.

Enough Was Enough!

Dottie was mad. She knew her husband was not getting his medications on time. She was ready to complain.

Her husband, Leonard, who was a diabetic, had been admitted two days earlier because he could not get his blood sugar under control. Nobody really said what the problem was; all they did was check his blood sugar and give him insulin.

Dottie had not seen a doctor go near her husband since they got there. The nurses came and went but never seemed to know what was going on. Leonard's medicines were different, including his insulin, and he wasn't being given any of his medications at the right time. Now he had to get up to go to the bathroom, and no one was coming to help!

Dottie went to the information area on the main floor and asked to speak to someone about filing a complaint. She was directed to the patient representative's office. The patient representative took down the information Dottie gave her and agreed to speak to someone about it and get back to her by the end of the day.

A few hours later, the patient representative came to find Dottie and Leonard. She said she had done some checking and that Leonard's doctor and an endocrinologist (a doctor who specialized in treating diabetes) had been in to see Leonard earlier that day before Dottie had arrived. The specialist had changed Leonard's insulin as well as the times of the doses. The nurses were testing the blood sugars more frequently and reporting those to the doctor. The doctor was watching Leonard's blood sugars very closely to be sure the new insulin was working as planned. If everything went as expected, and Leonard's blood sugars stayed in the normal range, he would be going home on a new insulin regimen.

The patient representative had also spoken with the nursing supervisor. The nursing supervisor told the representative that they were short staffed and they were trying to get to all of their patients as soon as possible. The nursing supervisor recommended that Dottie call the nurse's station at least ten minutes before she actually needed help getting Leonard to the bathroom.

Dottie felt better. She still worried about Leonard, but at least she knew the staff was doing their job in handling his care.

R_xpert Advice

Before you file a complaint, do the following:

➢ Obtain a copy of your hospital's Patient Bill of Rights. This may be included in the packet of information that you received on admission. Know your rights before you complain, and target a specific right in your complaint.

➢ Take action! The fear of retaliation by hospital staff towards a patient or family member who complains often causes people not to file a complaint. File the complaint and get the proper care for you or your loved one.

➢ State the facts in a clear and concise way. State who was involved, what happened, when it happened, where it happened, how it happened, and why you think it happened. File the complaint while all of the facts are still fresh in your mind.[19]

Try to resolve the complaint within the hospital

➤ If this is a complaint against a specific nursing station or unit, give the nursing staff the benefit of the doubt and the opportunity to make it up to you. Try to resolve the complaint with the nurse manager directly. If the nurse manager does not resolve the issue, then go to the nursing supervisor; if the supervisor fails to resolve your complaint, take it to the vice president of nursing.

➤ If your complaint is related to a hospital-wide issue, such as cleanliness or hazardous conditions, first go to the patient representative. If the patient representative does not resolve the complaint, go to the risk manager, and if the complaint is not resolved, go to the chief operating officer. Your last resort would be to go to the chief executive officer of the hospital.

If you feel the hospital is providing an insufficient quality of care, and you feel the need to file a complaint with an outside organization, you have several options.

➤ State agencies: You can file a complaint against a hospital in your state. Look up the contact information for the Department of Health and request information regarding filing a complaint.

➤ Medicare Complaint Program: If you are a Medicare beneficiary, you can file a complaint by contacting the Quality Improvement Organization (QIO) in your state.

➤ The Joint Commission on the Accreditation of Healthcare Organizations (JCAHO) is a national hospital accrediting organization. The JCAHO anonymously reviews all quality-of-care complaints (not billing complaints). The easiest way to submit a complaint is by e-mail: complaint@jcaho.org.You can also submit a complaint at www.jointcommision. org. For information on the complaint process, call 1-800-994-6610.

Bottom Line

Know the steps to file a complaint and get the results you want. First file the complaint internally within the hospital, and if you do not get the resolution you need, file the complaint with an outside organization.

Safety Tip #43
Prevent Discharge Disasters:
What You Should Know before
Leaving the Hospital

You're going home. It is the time you've been waiting for. You're tired of being poked and prodded and eating hospital food. The doctor has released you, and now you are free to go. Before you dart out the door, there's something very important you need to know.

Serious medication errors and oversights can happen in the process of being discharged from the hospital. What's worse, these errors could put you right back in the hospital. Take a few steps to ensure that you have all of the necessary information about your medications and follow-up care before you leave the hospital.

Ready to Go!

At 8:00 a.m., Aggie's doctor had come in to see her. He told her that she would be going home that day. At 8:15 a.m., Aggie was dressed, packed, and ready to go. She sat on the side of the bed with her purse in her lap, waiting for her daughter to pick her up. Little did Aggie know that it would be several hours before she was ready to leave the hospital. There was still a lot to do.

Aggie's daughter, Joann, came in to see her mom and prepare to take her home. Joann knew that there was a lot of information that she needed first. Joann did not let her mom pressure her to go. She took out a pad of paper with several questions on it and plenty of room to write down all of the information the doctor, pharmacist, and nurses gave her.

The pharmacist came to Aggie's room to give her a list of all the medications she would be taking at home. This list included fifteen different medications to treat a variety of conditions, including high blood pressure, heart failure, diabetes, thyroid dysfunction, pain, and constipation.

The pharmacist sat down with Joann and Aggie and reviewed each medication including the name of the drug, what it was for, how Aggie should take it, and possible side effects. The pharmacist gave Joann the med list and asked Joann to repeat the information back to him so he could be sure they understood the directions.

Joann still had some questions. She asked the pharmacist if certain drugs could be taken together to help simplify her mom's regimen. She also asked which drugs to take with or without food. Joann asked if her mom should avoid anything, like her evening glass of wine or certain fruit juices. She asked what to do if her mom had a side effect from any of the drugs. Last, she asked if her mom should stop taking any of her old medications she still had at home. Joann wanted to get as much information as possible to help prevent problems later on.

Joann and Aggie left the hospital with information about the medications and follow-up care. They also had phone numbers for the doctor, pharmacist, and nurse in case they had additional questions.

R_xpert Advice

➢ Before leaving the hospital, ask for written instructions about your follow-up care and your medications. Be sure that you understand these instructions.

➢ Be sure to get an updated, written list of medication from the nurse or pharmacist. These should be the medications you will be taking once you get home.

➢ Review the med list with the nurse or pharmacist, and be sure you understand what the medications are for and how to take them, and any possible side effects. If you are not able to do this, have your caregiver review the list of medications with the pharmacist or nurse.

➤ Ask your caregiver or advocate to be there with you when you are discharged from the hospital. Your caregiver or advocate will help by asking questions that may not occur to you. Ask your caregiver to bring a pad of paper and a pen to write down all of the important discharge information.

➤ Make sure you find out which of your old medications you will be taking and which ones you can throw out.

➤ Ask if you should avoid combining with your medications with any over-the-counter drugs, vitamins, supplements, or herbal products. Many of these products can cause serious reactions with prescription medications, so ask your pharmacist first.

➤ Many drugs, including pain medications and sleeping pills, interact with alcohol and should not be taken together. Ask if there are any foods or drinks, including alcoholic beverages, that you should avoid while taking these medications.

➤ Ask about side effects. Find out what you should do if you have a side effect. Symptoms of side effects include excessive drowsiness, nausea, vomiting, diarrhea, and so on. Call your doctor if you are experiencing a side effect.

➤ Get your prescriptions filled as soon as possible after leaving the hospital. Prevent serious errors by starting your new meds right away.

Bottom Line

Before you leave the hospital, ask for written instructions and speak with your nurse, doctor, and pharmacist about your medications and follow-up care. Be sure you understand these instructions and follow them closely to prevent a rapid return to your hospital bed.

Part 5

Play It Safe:
Preventing Medication Errors at Home

You're Not Home Free!

Once you've left the doctor's office or hospital with your new prescriptions, it's up to you to get them filled and take them correctly. This is no easy chore. Sometimes, due to high cost, lack of insurance coverage, or other factors, people do not get their prescriptions filled. Other patients pick up their medications, yet fail to take them or fail to take them correctly due to confusing directions, complex medication regimens, uncomfortable side effects, and a host of other reasons.

The following safety tips will give you "tried and true" strategies for helping you to take your medications correctly and avoid dangerous medication errors at home.

Safety Tip #44
Take as Directed: Easier
Said than Done

Although it seems obvious that not taking your medications the way your doctor told you to is a dangerous mistake that could lead to serious problems, many people continue to do this. They may not take enough medication, take too much, take it at the wrong time, or just not take it at all. Some people fear having a side effect or a bad reaction and some just don't have the money to pay for their drugs. Whatever the reason, not taking your medications correctly may lead to serious problems. There are many resources to help you take your medications correctly. Ask your doctor or pharmacist and read this story.

Don't Just Stop

Peggy knew she had high blood pressure, and her doctor had prescribed a "blood pressure pill," but frankly, she never noticed a difference whether she took it or not, so when the prescription ran out, she just stopped taking it.

A few weeks later, Peggy was having terrible headaches and she was dizzy and lightheaded. She knew something was not right, so she called her doctor.

The doctor examined Peggy and took her blood pressure. It was 152/96, which was high. The doctor asked Peggy if she was taking her amlodipine, the blood pressure pill, every day like she was supposed to. Peggy admitted to the doctor that she had stopped taking it several weeks before. She told him that she never saw a difference, so she stopped it. The doctor told Peggy that not taking the medicine was causing her high blood pressure, headaches, and dizziness. He told her to start taking the amlodipine again and check her blood pressure every day. He explained that despite not feeling any effects of the medication, it was actually saving her life.

Peggy had not realized not taking this medication could lead to such serious consequences. She put the "blood pressure pill" back in her pillbox and started to take it every day.

R_xpert Advice

> ➤ Take your medications as prescribed by your doctor. Never stop taking a drug unless your doctor tells you to do so.

> ➤ Ask your pharmacist for help in creating a medication schedule, one that fits well with your daily routine and is easy for you to remember.

> ➤ Get a pillbox to help you to remember to take your pills as directed.

> ➤ Ask your pharmacist if it is safe to take certain medications together at the same time of day.

> ➤ Ask your pharmacist about any side effects and what to do if you have a side effect.

> ➤ Ask your doctor or pharmacist to explain the importance of taking your prescriptions. Even though you may not notice a difference at first, not taking them can lead to serious problems.

Bottom Line

Take all of your medications as prescribed even if you don't feel that the drug is doing anything. Not taking them can lead to serious consequences.

Safety Tip #45
Have a Plan: Create a
Medication Schedule

Throughout the course of this book, I have discussed the importance of keeping a medication list. Just as important is keeping a medication schedule. A medication schedule is a checklist of all of your drugs and the times that you take them.

Having a medication schedule helps you and your caregiver stay organized and serves as a guide to help you remember when to take your pills. It also helps when you or your caregiver is filling your pillbox. Having a medication schedule is especially important for those who take several different drugs at different times of day.

Too Many Pills

Jim left the doctor's office with a fistful of new prescriptions. His doctor had just prescribed four new drugs for him, which put the total number of prescriptions that he was taking at eight different pills every day. Some were to be taken in the morning, some in the afternoon, and others at night. How was he going to keep this straight?

Jim went to the pharmacy to have the prescriptions filled. He asked the pharmacist for help. In addition to asking the names of the drugs and what they were used for, Jim made it a point to ask exactly how he should take them. Could he take the new pills at the same time he took the ones he was taking already? He didn't want to be taking pills all day long.

The pharmacist told him exactly how and when to take the new pills, taking into consideration that Jim already took pills in the morning and at bedtime. The pharmacist was able to work with Jim to create a medication schedule that would work for him.

Jim was pleased. He had received helpful information from the pharmacist and was now able to take all of his medications as prescribed by his doctor on a convenient dosing schedule. Jim felt better already!

R$_x$pert Advice

> The medications schedule is a chart that lists the drugs you are taking, what they do, what they look like, and the time of day that you take them. It helps you and your caregiver to keep track of your meds and to take them correctly.

> Ask your pharmacist for help when filling out your medication schedule. Your pharmacist may be able to consolidate the times you take your meds to make taking your medication safer and easier.

> Show your medication schedule to your doctors and other health-care providers to ensure they all know how and when you are taking your medications.

Bottom Line

Ask your pharmacist for help if you need to create a medication schedule. He or she is there to provide the information you need to take your medications safely and correctly.

Bonus

Go to www.drmarysue.com to download a free Medication Schedule.

Safety Tip #46
Simple Solutions to Help You Remember to Take Your Medication

Missing doses, taking your meds late, or taking an overdose are just some of the medication errors that can result from improper medication management. Learning how to manage your meds and taking them correctly will help to prevent potentially fatal medication errors from happening to you. If you have ever taken prescription medications, chances are you have missed a dose or, at times, forgotten to take them completely. It's easy to forget, especially when you are busy or distracted. It doesn't matter if you take only one pill a day or several, if you are young and alert or if you are elderly and forgetful, remembering to take your meds is difficult, but there are ways to make it easier.

"I Only Take My Pills When I Remember"

Jim was out of town for an important business meeting, and he was late. As he was hurrying to the cab, he felt his heart start to pound quickly. He was having trouble catching his breath, and his head began pounding too. Jim thought that the stress of all of the travel was starting to take its toll. He just needed to get this meeting over with and everything would be okay.

Jim arrived at the office for the meeting, but he felt horrible. The headache was getting worse—he couldn't think straight and his chest was pounding. He asked the secretary for some water and sat down on the couch. The next thing Jim knew, he was in an ambulance on his way to the hospital. The secretary had called 9-1-1 when Jim had missed the couch and fallen to the floor.

The emergency room doctor asked Jim what medications he was taking. Jim took two pills. He did not know the name of them, he just knew they were for high blood pressure. The doctor asked Jim if he had taken the pills that day, and Jim replied, "I only take them when I remember." It had been at least a week since he had taken them. He never noticed any difference whether he took them or not, and he had an especially difficult time remembering when he was on the road.

The doctor told Jim that he had passed out because his blood pressure had become dangerously high since he had not taken his medications every day like his doctor had prescribed. He told Jim to get organized and take his pills daily like he was supposed to. He told Jim to get a pillbox and put one pill in each compartment for every day of the week. That way he would know at a glance whether or not he had taken a pill that day. He also told Jim to take his medication at the same time every day and to schedule it along with something else that he did routinely, like brush his teeth or eat breakfast.

Jim took the doctor's advice to heart. He got the pillbox from the pharmacy and put a week's worth of pills in it. This would help him stay organized. Still, he knew it would be tough to remember to take his pills, especially while he was away from home, so he programmed his smart phone with a daily alarm which he set to remind him to take his pills. He was never without his smart phone.

He then took it one-step further and programmed a daily alert in his computer, which would also remind him to take his pills. Last, Jim made a list of his medications. He put the name of the drugs, how he took them, and any medication allergies on a med list. Then he put this list in his wallet. He also put this information on his smart phone, just to be sure.

R$_x$pert Advice

Staying organized is the key to medication management. However, this can be overwhelming especially if you take many different medications. Here are some pointers to help:

➤ Read the prescription label. You may think that you know how to take your medications, but check the label for any information that may be confusing and unclear. If you are confused about how to take a medication, call the pharmacist first.

➢ Make sure you understand the directions on the label. Sometimes, you might read the label, but still not know what to do. Confusing directions can lead to serious problems when the medication is taken incorrectly.

➢ Check the refill information before you actually need the refill. If you wait too long and there are no refills left, you may run out of pills and go for days without your medication. Your doctor needs to authorize a refill before the pharmacist can fill it. This may take several days. Your pharmacist can help you with refills, but you need to call in advance to allow plenty of time.

➢ Keep an updated list of your medications. This is the easiest way to stay organized. The medication list is where you will write in the names of all of your drugs, how you take them, and any side effects. It also has a place to write in your allergies. The med list should include all prescriptions as well as over-the-counter, herbal, dietary supplements, natural products, vitamins, etc., that you may be taking. Ask your pharmacist if you need help filling out your med list.

➢ Create a medication-dosing schedule. Keep a medication dosing schedule that lists all of the medications you take, how you take them, and when you take them. If you need help filling this out, ask your pharmacist for help.

➢ Make taking your pills part of your daily routine. For example, if you take your pills in the morning, make it a habit to take them after brushing your teeth or after eating your breakfast. Just be sure to match up the routines with the proper way to take the drugs. Some medications must not be taken together, with food, or at certain times. Your pharmacist can help you coordinate your medication schedule with your routines.

➢ For medication that is stored in the refrigerator, put a sticky note on the refrigerator door that says "Take Meds."

➢ If you take a medication with a meal, put the bottle near you on the table where you eat and be sure to take your pill when you finish eating. If you leave your pill bottles out in the open and you have small children around, be sure to put your pill bottles away in a locked cabinet when you're done.

➢ Set an alarm to signal when it is time to take your pills. Then be sure to take the medications when the alarm goes off. Don't ignore it.

➢ Keep a daily pillbox. The daily pillbox has separate compartments for each day of the week to help you stay organized and remember if you took your pills that day. Pillboxes come with varying numbers of compartments for different times of day (morning, noon, evening, and bedtime) and in different sizes to accommodate many different medication combinations, shapes, and sizes. Many pharmacies supply pillboxes at no charge. The major drawback to using pillboxes is that they are not childproof. Leaving the pillbox where a child could reach it can lead to accidental poisonings. Be sure to put it in a locked cabinet when children are in the house.

➢ Try a pill reminder gadget. These days, you can find many different types of gadgets to help you remember to take your pills. These range from simple alarms and voice reminders to automatic, lockable, pill dispensers. Some of the more advanced devices are expensive, but the cost may be offset by the peace of mind from knowing you are taking your medications correctly.

➢ For those who are computer savvy or have a smart phone, you may want to use technology to help you take your meds on time. If you are on the computer for much of the day, you can set a computer-generated alert (like an electronic sticky note) to help you remember. You can also use your cell phone to set an alarm that will go off at a certain time each day or set cell phone calendars with recurring reminders to take your meds.

➢ Ask for help. Caregivers are a critical asset in helping you remember to take your meds. They can help you with your medication schedule and help you fill your pillbox. They can design a set routine for you and place your meds where you will see them.

Bottom Line

Staying organized is the key to taking your medications correctly. Pick any one of the above solutions to help you take your meds as prescribed.

Safety Tip #47
Med Minder Miracles!
Talking Pillboxes, Glowing
Bottle Caps, and More

These days there are about as many different gadgets on the market to remind you to take your medications as there are ways to forget. Whether you want to spend a lot or a little, you can find a number of ways to help you take your medications on time.

"I Can't Remember if I Took My Pills"

Henry was always forgetting to take his pills. He felt that all he did all day was take pills, and he did not like it one bit. His daughter, Penny, got angry with him every time she found out he had not taken his pills. He did not know what to do.

Penny knew she had to do something. Her dad's health was getting worse, and she knew it was because he kept forgetting to take his meds. One time, he forgot to take them for three days, and another time he'd forgotten that he had already taken his medicine and then took twice the prescribed dose.

Penny found an automatic pill dispenser with an alarm. She decided to buy one of these for her dad and see if it helped. Several weeks after Penny had bought the automatic dispenser, her dad said that he felt the best he had in years, and she noticed that he was more alert and attentive. He said that he had not missed a dose of his medications in the past few weeks, ever since she had bought him the new machine.

Henry's daughter was glad she invested in the automatic pill dispenser. Her dad was feeling better, and she finally had some peace of mind that he was taking his pills as prescribed.

R_xpert Advice

Here is a partial list of great gadgets you can use to help remember to take your medications.

> *Automatic Pill Dispensers:* Automatic electronic pill dispensers are convenient medication organizers that come with an alarm to remind a person to take their medications on time. The machine dispenses the correct dose at the appropriate time. Many of these automatic pill dispensers are equipped with locks, so the person taking the pills cannot overdose. The caregiver loads and programs the dispenser, and some will even notify the caregiver if a pill is missed. Some dispensers need to be refilled weekly, others every two weeks, and others on a monthly basis. Some dispensers alert a person to take their pills one to two times a day, while others will alert up to four times a day. Prices for the basic organizer with a timer start around $30. The more advanced models go for approximately $150.

> Some fancier models record the time a pill was taken, display how often the pills were taken, and then provide this information to caregivers and doctors. These pillboxes will even send an e-mail, text message, or phone call to notify a remote caregiver if a med dose has been missed. These pillboxes are high-end and charge a monthly subscription fee.

> *Alarm Wristwatches:* The alarm wristwatch is a nifty gadget that sets off an alarm when it is time to take your medications. You may program alarms to go off several times a day and set the alert for audio, vibrating, or even a text message (which is especially helpful if you are away from home). Many of the watches also have room to store important medical information,

such as medical history, allergies, blood type, and insurance information. The alarm wristwatches range in price from $30 to $100 depending on the features you want.

➤ *Prescription Bottle Caps with Alarms:* You can set the alarm right on your prescription bottle with a special bottle cap that fits onto a standard prescription bottle. The alarm sounds when it is time to take your pills. Some caps include visual alerts like flashing lights or displays. Some caps even trigger an alert when you haven't taken your pills and will call you on your cell phone to remind you. *Warning:* many of these prescription bottle caps are not childproof. Ask your pharmacist before you use these caps if you have children around the house.

➤ *"There's an app for that":* For the tech savvy, you can find plenty of software applications to help remind you to take your meds. You can use these apps can on your personal home computer, your smart phone or PDA, and even your office PC.

Many of these programs include daily alarms that beep, send a text message on your computer screen, or even e-mail you. The software includes neat features like medication lists, medication dosing schedules, a log of how often you took your medication (or missed it), and prescription refill reminders.

Many of these software programs are free, and some come with a monthly subscription fee. When you find one you like, check it out first to be sure there are no hidden costs and that your medical information will be secure.

Bottom Line

There are many different types of medication reminder gadgets on the market today. Prices range according to the included features. Be sure to select the one(s) that best suit your health-care needs or the needs of your family.

Bonus

Go to www.drmarysue.com to see new and nifty gadgets to help you take your medications correctly.

Safety Tip #48
"Oops! I Did It Again!" What to Do if You Miss a Dose

Generally, if you miss a scheduled dose of your medication, take the missed dose as soon as you remember to take it, unless it is near the time to take the next scheduled dose. In that case, skip the missed dose and resume your usual dosing schedule at the time you normally take your medication. Still, be sure to ask your pharmacist what to do regarding missed doses for each of your medications, as recommendations may differ from drug to drug. Whatever you do, do not double up to make up for missed doses. When in doubt, contact your doctor or pharmacist for instructions if you have missed a dose.

Getting It Together

Leslie just couldn't get it together. As a mother of four kids, she was constantly running around, getting up early, staying up late, and never paying attention to her own health. Leslie had diabetes. She was supposed to take glyburide, one pill every day to help keep her blood sugar under control. Unfortunately, she rarely remembered to take it. She just always seemed to forget. When she did remember, she doubled up and took two pills at once to make up for any doses she missed.

During her checkup, her doctor noticed that Leslie's blood sugar was high. He asked Leslie how she was taking her diabetes medication. Leslie admitted that taking pills was not something that she was good at. She was always forgetting. When she did remember, she took two to make up for any missed doses. The doctor was not happy. He told Leslie that it was critical that she start to take her diabetes drugs as prescribed, one pill every day at the same time. This would help to keep her blood sugar under control. The more concerning issue for the doctor was that Leslie was doubling up on her doses. Taking double the amount of the drug could lower Leslie's blood sugar to a dangerous level, causing a headache, shakiness, or trouble concentrating. She may even pass out, and with four small children to take care of this could be extremely dangerous.

Her doctor recommended that she get a pillbox and place it where she would remember to take her medication every day. Leslie had no idea that not taking her medications as prescribed was so dangerous. She had learned her lesson. From now on, no matter how busy she got, she would take care of herself first. Her health and her family depended on it.

R&pert Advice

> If you forget to take your medications, try to take them at the same time as you routinely do something else, like brushing your teeth or getting ready for bed. Placing the pillbox near your toothbrush will help you to remember not to forget your pills.

> If you tend to forget your pills and leave for work, it would be a good idea to carry an extra dose of your medications with you. Ask your pharmacist for a labeled prescription bottle with a childproof cap to carry with you.

> You may find a medication reminder system helpful if you frequently forget to take your medications.

> Create and keep a medication schedule. This will help you to remember when to take your medications.

Bottom Line

If you miss a dose, take the missed dose as soon as you remember, unless it is almost time for the next scheduled dose. In that case, skip the missed dose and resume your normal schedule with the next dose.

When in doubt, contact your doctor or pharmacist for instructions if you have missed or doubled up a dose of your medication.

Bonus

Go to www.drmarysue.com to see several types of medication reminder systems and download a Medication Schedule.

Safety Tip #49
Overdose? Don't Hesitate! Get Help

Read this information before an emergency happens and keep the Poison Control number handy.

If you suspect that there has been a drug overdose by an adult or child, read the label on the bottle for any emergency first aid information and act on it. Next, call the Poison Control Center.

Poison Control Center Number: 1-800-222-1222

(American Association of Poison Control Centers)

Don't Wait. Get Emergency Help Fast.

The National Poison Control Center (1-800-222-1222) can be called from anywhere in the United States. This national number will let you talk to experts in poisoning. They will give you further instructions.

This is a free and confidential service. You should call if you have any questions about poisoning or poison prevention. It does *not* need to be an emergency. You can call for any reason, twenty-four hours a day, seven days a week.

Drug Overdose

A drug overdose means that you have taken or given more than the safe dose of a drug. Accidental overdose can result from taking the wrong dose when a person does not read the prescription label or the directions on an over-the-counter (OTC) drug. An overdose may also happen if a person does not understand how to take the medication. A drug overdose can happen to adults, but it is also common among small children whose parents do not understand how to accurately measure the drug and accidentally give too much of the medication

Many people think that over-the-counter drugs like acetaminophen, aspirin, ibuprofen, decongestants, antihistamines, iron pills, vitamins, supplements, and diet pills are harmless, but if there is an overdose, the results can be fatal.

R$_x$pert Advice

If you suspect an overdose, call the Poison

Control Center at 1-800-222-1222.

> ➢ Before you need it, find out how to contact your local poison control center and keep the information handy for emergencies. To find your local center and phone number go to www.drugs.com/poison-control.html.

Follow these precautions to prevent an accidental drug overdose.

> ➢ Read the label on the prescription bottle or the over-the-counter medication bottle or package and be certain that you understand the directions before taking it or giving it to a child. If you are not 100 percent certain that you know how to take or give the medication, call your pharmacist for help.

> ➢ Never take or give more of the medication than the doctor tells you. Never take more over-the-counter medication than is stated in the product directions, even if it seems fine.

> ➢ Learn the difference between a teaspoon (tsp) and a tablespoon (tbsp). A teaspoon is the smaller spoon and generally holds 5 ml (or 5 cc). A tablespoon is the larger

spoon and generally holds 15 ml (or 15 cc). However, different teaspoons and tablespoons may hold different amounts and could lead to an overdose of a liquid medication, so use the dosage cup provided with liquid medicines to measure an exact dose.

➢ If a cup, dropper, syringe, or any other medication measuring device comes with the drug (prescription and over-the-counter), use it to accurately measure the medication. This is a safe and convenient way to prevent a drug overdose.

➢ Know the main ingredient in the over-the-counter (OTC) medications you take. Many OTC products contain the same active ingredients but are packaged differently. You may be taking or giving double or even triple the dose of the exact same medication.

➢ Sometimes, children are better at opening "childproof" bottles than adults are. Store medications out of out of reach of children just to be safe.

Bottom Line

Read the label on the prescription bottle or over-the-counter package and follow the directions, being sure to use the correct measuring device. Call your doctor or poison control center immediately if you suspect a drug overdose.

Safety Tip #50
"But I Only Took Some Tylenol."
How to Avoid a Tylenol Overdose

If you are the type of person who goes "all out" even when you are in pain, listen up! I am about to tell you something that may save your life.

Tylenol (aka acetaminophen) is a very popular pain reliever. Millions of people use Tylenol every day to treat pain and reduce fever, and it's safe and effective when used properly.

What most people don't know is that if you take too much Tylenol, it can be deadly. Tylenol in overdose amounts can seriously damage your liver and, if left untreated for even a short time, may shut your liver down completely and you may require a liver transplant to save your life.

"It Was Just Tylenol"

Matt's back was killing him. He had hurt it in a skiing accident a week ago and the doctor had prescribed two pain meds for him. One of the pain meds was Vicodin and the directions were to take one to two tablets every four to six hours as needed for moderate pain. The label said not to exceed eight tablets a day. He also got some Percocet and was supposed to take one tablet every six hours if needed for severe pain.

These two pain meds were not to be taken together. Matt decided to take both meds since he thought that would help him get back on his feet sooner. In addition to the prescription drugs, Matt had a bottle of extra-strength Tylenol, and he was taking two of those every eight hours. It was just Tylenol—what could go wrong?

After a few days of taking these medications together, Matt started to feel lousy. He lost his appetite and his stomach started to hurt. He felt like throwing up and he was sweating. He called his friend who took him to the emergency room. The doctor asked Matt what medications he was taking, and Matt told him that he was taking Vicodin and Percocet and extra-strength Tylenol. The doctor knew that each one of these medications contained acetaminophen, and when he added up the total amount of acetaminophen, he figured that Matt was taking more than double the safe dose! Matt was having symptoms of acetaminophen overdose. The doctor treated Matt for the overdose and told him he was very lucky. Had he not come into the emergency room when he did, he could have had a liver failure.

Matt had no idea that taking too much acetaminophen could cause so much harm. He learned the hard way that more is not better. From now on, he would take his prescription medications as directed and ask for advice from his pharmacist before taking over-the-counter drugs.

R_xpert Advice

> Acetaminophen is an ingredient found in many prescription painkillers and over-the-counter analgesics (pain relievers) and cold products. It may be labeled as acetaminophen, Tylenol, or even APAP. Be sure you know if there is acetaminophen and how much is in each of the products you are taking.

> For an adult, doses over 4000 mg of acetaminophen a day is too much. This is equal to taking twelve regular-strength tablets of Tylenol or eight extra-strength tablets over a twenty-four-hour period.

> If you take acetaminophen with alcoholic beverages, the risk of liver damage increases. If you consistently consume three or more alcoholic drinks a day, your maximum dose of acetaminophen is just 2000 mg a day, or one-half the normal recommended dose.

➤ Ask your pharmacist if your prescription or over-the-counter pain reliever contains acetaminophen.

➤ Do not take more than one drug that contains acetaminophen at a time.

➤ Ask your doctor or pharmacist if you have questions about your over-the-counter or prescription medications and do not take more than the prescribed dose.

➤ If you suspect a Tylenol (acetaminophen) overdose, do not wait; call the National Poison Control Center (1-800-222-1222) or your doctor for further instructions.

Bottom Line

People think that over-the-counter drugs are "safe," but they can be just as dangerous as prescription drugs if not taken correctly.

Safety Tip #51
OTC Is Still a Drug: Read the Label on Over-the-Counter (OTC) Medications

It may seem basic, but many people do not read the label on an over-the-counter drug package. Just because a drug is available at the drugstore or grocery store without a prescription does not mean that it is completely safe to use. In fact, many of the drugs that are available over-the-counter today were once available by prescription only. Over-the-counter drugs are still *drugs*. They can be just as dangerous as prescription drugs if not taken correctly.

Too Drowsy to Drive

Angie was getting ready for bed. She took her prescription sleeping pill, and since she felt a headache coming on, she decided to take some Advil. Angie had some Advil PM, so she took that for the headache. The next morning, Angie was still very tired and was unable to wake up. She had never felt this groggy after taking her sleeping pill before. She wondered what could be wrong.

Angie called her pharmacist to ask what could be the matter. She told the pharmacist that she had taken some Advil PM with her prescription sleeping pill the night before. Could this be what was causing her to be so drowsy?

The pharmacist told Angie that Advil PM contained two different drugs in one pill. It contained one drug for pain and one drug for sleep. The drug in the Advil PM had intensified the effect of the prescription sleeping pill, causing Angie to be very sleepy the next morning. The pharmacist told her that she should always read the information on the Advil PM and other over-the-counter drug labels, since many OTC products can interact with prescription drugs.

Since Angie was too drowsy to drive, she stayed home from work that day. From now on, to be safe, she would always check with her pharmacist before taking any over-the-counter drugs with her prescription medications.

R_xpert Advice

➤ Read the information on the label of the over-the-counter (OTC) bottle or package. This includes information about how to take the product, drug interactions, and side effects.

➤ Be certain that you understand the information on the OTC package. If you do not understand, ask your pharmacist to explain it to you.

➤ Ask your pharmacist if the OTC medication will interact with any of the prescription medications you are taking. Many drug interactions lead to serious effects like excessive drowsiness or dizziness.

➤ Ask your pharmacist what side effects to expect with the OTC medication, and what to do if you have a side effect.

➤ Ask your pharmacist if there is anything that you need to avoid like driving or drinking alcoholic beverages while taking the OTC medication.

➤ Identify the active ingredients in the OTC product. Check your other prescription medications and ask your pharmacist if they contain the same or very similar drug product as the OTC med.

➤ OTC products like ibuprofen, naproxen, or aspirin contain anti-inflammatory drugs for pain relief. If you also take a prescription for pain like Celebrex, diclofenac, Fiorinal, indomethacin, or others, you may be taking more pain medication than you need.

➤ Do not take more than one over-the-counter product with the same active ingredient in it. For example, do not take more than one product containing acetaminophen or aspirin as this may lead to a dangerous overdose.

> ➤ Use OTC products that contain only one drug. Avoid OTC products that treat multiple symptoms and contain several different medications. You may not need all of those medications, and you could have a reaction or side effect to any of the drugs in the product.

> ➤ Do not take more than the recommended dose. Do not take the product more often than the label recommends.

> ➤ When giving OTC medication to children, be especially careful about how much you are giving them. Use the measuring cup or spoon that comes with the product so you can give the exact amount to a child. Kitchen teaspoons do not measure the exact amount (5 ml). If necessary, use a measuring spoon (teaspoon) to get the exact amount. Serious overdoses have happened when parents have given their babies the wrong dose of an OTC medication.

> ➤ Never give children OTC products meant for adults. Use only those products specifically made for children and dosed by their age or weight.

> ➤ Check the expiration date on the box or bottle. Using expired meds can be harmful. Properly dispose of any unused or expired over-the-counter meds.

Bottom Line

Just because a drug is available over the counter does not mean it is safe to take. Drug interactions, side effects, and other bad reactions can happen. Read the label and ask your doctor or pharmacist if you have any questions about how to take your over-the-counter medications safely.

Bonus

Go to www.drmarysue.com for instructions on how to read the label on an OTC product.

Safety Tip #52
"The Granny Syndrome"

Accidental, pediatric drug poisonings are extremely dangerous, sometimes lethal, events. One of the most common ways children accidentally get ahold of dangerous drugs is from Grandma's purse.

This phenomenon is so common that we in the medical community call it "The Granny Syndrome," i.e. poisonings resulting from grandparents' medications that are taken by small children when these medications are left within reach.[20]

Keep out of Reach of Children

Amber, an eighteen-month-old handful of action and energy, was bright, resourceful, curious, and a natural explorer. She was double-trouble now that she could walk.

Amber's mom and dad wanted a date night, so Amber's grandmother agreed to babysit. As soon as she arrived, Grandma laid her big purse down by the front door and went into the kitchen to get some last-minute instructions from Amber's mom.

As few minutes later, Grandma noticed that it was very quiet. Amber must be up to something. To her astonishment and horror, Grandma found the contents of her purse spilled all around, and Amber sitting on the floor in the middle of it. Amber was in the process of tearing open the plastic bag where Grandma kept her heart pills. Grandma jumped up and snatched the plastic bag from Amber. Had she come in just one minute later, Amber may have opened the bag and taken the pills.

Grandma was shaken up and felt guilty about being so careless with her purse. She knew it had medications in it, but she did not realize that Amber had become so fast and so inquisitive.

Grandma learned her lesson the hard way. Never again would she carry her medications in a plastic bag that Amber could easily open. She would find a lockable pillbox for her medications, and she would keep that purse out of Amber's reach.

R$_x$pert Advice

As a grandparent, parent, or caregiver of small children, there are many things that you can and should do to prevent accidental poisonings.

➢ Keep medications in a locked cabinet out of reach of children. Parents, grandparents, and caregivers must know that any drug that is stored in the proximity of the child is a potential threat. Many poisonings happen when medications are left within reach of small children on low-lying tables, countertops, cabinets, or shelves. Any area that is within three feet from the floor or placed anywhere near the child is "easy access."

➢ A child-resistant bottle cap is not enough protection. Childproof your home and keep drugs away from locations where your child plays.

➢ Make sure that all caregivers know the phone number for the National Poison Control Center and call it immediately if they suspect there has been a poisoning. The number is 1-800-222-1222.

➢ Keep the Poison Control Center on speed dial or in your cell phone.

➢ Never leave a pill bottle or container that is not child-resistant in your purse. Store your pills in child-resistant pill bottles and in a locked cabinet.

➢ Child-resistant does not mean "childproof." Many children are able to open these bottles, and thousands of accidental poisonings happen each year when children get ahold of and take medications that were stored in child-resistant pill bottles.

➤ Watch out for topical patches and gels, including nitroglycerin patches for the heart, fentanyl patches for severe pain, testosterone patches, and even the nicotine patch. Discarded patches sitting in the wastebasket still have active medication in them and can cause poisoning. Children have been known to pull the patch right off of an adult's arm and begin to suck on it, so be vigilant.

➤ Topical gels also pose a risk of poisoning. Grandfathers who use testosterone gel can inadvertently transfer the gel from their skin to a toddler sitting on their lap without even knowing they are causing harm. If you are wearing topical gel and holding a child, wear a long-sleeved shirt.

➤ Grandparents should carry an updated list of all their medications at all times. In the event that a child swallows your medications, you will need to know the name, strength, and purpose of the drugs.

➤ If you must carry a supply of medications with you, invest in a lockable pillbox. These look just like the weekly pillboxes, but they have a locking mechanism that will help to prevent accidental poisonings.

Childproof your home by taking precautions in three key areas of your home the kitchen, the bathroom, and all bedrooms.[21]

In the Kitchen

1) If you store medications in the kitchen, be sure they are stored in a high, locked cabinet, such as above your refrigerator. Just because medications are stored out of sight and out of reach of a child does not mean you are completely safe. Put a lock on the cabinet and make sure it stays locked at all times.

2) Never leave any pill bottles on the kitchen counter or in unlocked kitchen cabinets. It may be convenient for you, especially if you take your meds with meals, but be sure to put them away in the locked cabinet when you are done.

3) When you bring home medications from the grocery store or drugstore, be sure to unpack them first and put them away quickly and securely. Bright colored pills look like candy to a toddler, and they will try to eat them.

4) If you take a medication, like insulin, that must be stored in the refrigerator, use a lock on the refrigerator door.

5) Small children are prescribed amoxicillin and other antibiotics that must be kept in the refrigerator. The flavors, like bubblegum and grape, make it easier to give to a child, but may make the child think it is candy. Keep the bottle on a high shelf in the back of the refrigerator, out of a child's sight and reach.

6) If the phone rings or someone comes to the door while you are taking your pills, let the phone ring and return the call after you have taken your pills, the lids are tightly put back on, and the bottles are stored securely away. If you must go to the door, replace the lids, lock the pills in the cabinet, and then answer the door. Never leave pills unattended.

In the Bathroom

1) The "medicine cabinet" is not a safe place to store medications. Unless it is locked and out of a child's reach, it is not safe. Do not store medications there. Also, the heat and humidity from the bathtub or shower can easily break down your tablets and cause gelcaps to stick together.

2) Never store medications or other dangerous products under the bathroom sink. This includes liquids, creams, lotions, gels, vitamins, laxatives, and other products. This is too dangerous to risk. Put these products in a locked cabinet or locked closet.

3) Do not store your meds on top of the bathroom counter. Even over-the-counter drugs that you may feel are safe like vitamins, laxatives, allergy pills, and painkillers, are still potent medication and can cause severe harm to a child.

4) Get rid of any unused or expired meds before your small child comes for a visit. Clean out the bathroom cabinets and properly dispose of these unwanted drugs and take out the trash. Ask your pharmacist if there is a drug disposal program near you. See Safety Tip #57 for proper disposal of prescription drugs.

In the Bedroom

1) Remove all pill bottles from the top of the nightstand and the nightstand drawers. This includes bottles left behind by overnight guests.

2) Don't keep medicines on your dresser. A small child can easily use the drawers as steps to climb up and grab those pill bottles.

3) Check the floor and under the bed after you take your medication. Make sure you didn't drop a pill that can be found by an enterprising crawler.

4) If you store your medications on a high shelf in your bedroom closet, lock the closet door. Just because they are out of sight and up high does not mean that a child will not get to them.

In Addition to the Steps Above, Remember:

1) "Child-resistant" does not mean "childproof." Many parents know that their small, determined children can get the child-resistant cap off a prescription bottle faster than they can. Don't be fooled into a false sense of security.

2) Don't consolidate all of your pills into one prescription bottle. You could easily become confused and take the wrong pill, and if a child ingests medication from that bottle, you have no way of knowing which pills she took.

3) Don't take your pills in front of a small child. They will want to imitate you and take pills just like you.

Bottom Line

Nothing will stop a curious toddler from getting into your cupboards or purse. Take action to prevent an accidental poisoning from happening to a child you love.

Safety Tip #53
Generation Rx: Teen Abuse
of Prescription Drugs

Abuse of prescription drugs among teenagers has reached an alarming rate. The Partnership for a Drug-Free America has coined the term "generation Rx" for teens who intentionally abuse prescription drugs to get high.[22]

Prescription Drug Abuse—Not Only for Celebrities

Michael Jackson, Heath Ledger, Kurt Cobain, Chris Farley, Anna Nicole Smith, Brittany Murphy, River Phoenix, and Amy Winehouse—the list of celebrities who have died from prescription drug overdose continues to grow. However, it's not only celebrities who are abusing these drugs. Abuse of prescription drugs is second in popularity only to marijuana among teens ranging in age from twelve to seventeen years old. Adolescents most commonly abuse painkillers like OxyContin and Vicodin. However, Adderall and Ritalin also are abused at an alarming rate. Many teens and their parents mistakenly think that legal prescription drugs provide a "safer high" than illegal street drugs. However, they are dead wrong. Make the time to talk to your teenager about abusing prescription drugs and alcohol, and by using the names of the celebrities above, make sure your children realize they are playing a very dangerous game.

R_xpert Advice

One of the main reasons the abuse of prescription drugs among teenagers is so common, is that prescription drugs are so easy to get. Nearly one-third of new drug abusers say that their first time using drugs was with a prescription drug, specifically a painkiller. Almost two-thirds of the teens who have abused prescription drugs say they got them, bought them, or stole them from friends or relatives, and almost one-half of these teens say a relative or friend gave them prescription painkillers.[23] A family history of drug or alcohol abuse may predispose a teen to abuse drugs, but any teen could be at risk.

Here are a few warning signs that a teen you know may be abusing drugs.

- depression
- loss of interest in personal appearance or activities that used to bring enjoyment
- low self-esteem
- feeling that the teen does not fit in or is not popular
- sluggishness
- sleep disturbances
- aggressive or rebellious attitude toward authority figures
- difficulty paying attention
- shift in patterns of participation and attending social functions
- vague physical complaints that the teen indicates need to be treated by drugs or exaggeration of medical problems
- a family history of substance or alcohol abuse
- seeing multiple doctors and asking for prescriptions
- frequently borrowing money or having unexpected extra cash

As a parent, you can help to prevent teen abuse of prescription drugs by doing the following:

- talking and listening regularly to your teen
- being directly involved in your child's everyday world
- making it clear that you do not want him or her drinking or using drugs
- setting limits
- educating yourself about the risk of prescription drug abuse
- safeguarding your own prescription drugs—count and monitor your prescription drugs and keep them in a secure place

Bottom Line

Prescription drug abuse is not only for celebrities. Take time to talk to your teen about the dangers of abusing of prescription drugs.

Bonus

For more information about teenage prescription drug abuse go to www.drugfree.org.

Safety Tip #54
"Neither a Borrower nor a Lender Be"—Shakespeare

Borrowing someone else's prescription medication or lending someone your medications is extremely risky and dangerous. Don't do it. Borrowing or lending your meds can lead to an overdose, severe drug interactions, serious side effects, harmful allergic reactions—or all of the above.

Real Friends Don't Share Drugs

Dana was in a lot of pain. She had fallen off her mountain bike and hurt her knee. Her roommate, Kathy, had some Vicodin that she had taken the previous year for back pain, and she offered some to Dana.

Dana anxiously agreed to take them and then went to lie down. Two hours later, Dana woke up covered in a bright red, itchy rash, and she felt hot and sweaty. She was having trouble catching her breath. She called Kathy to come help her.

Dana was having an allergic reaction to the Vicodin. She knew that she was allergic to codeine, but she had never taken Vicodin before, and she did not know that it contained a form of codeine.

Kathy took Dana to the emergency room. The ER doctor treated her for the allergic reaction, and he gave Dana a pain medication for her knee that did not contain codeine.

R_xpert Advice

➢ Borrowing or lending medications is risky business. This can lead to serious side effects, drug interactions, and severe allergic reactions. Don't borrow pills from someone else. Call your doctor to get the medication that is right for you.

➢ Even though you may have good intentions, lending or sharing your medications with someone else can be harmful. When someone asks you for some of your pills, suggest they see their own doctor for help.

➢ Many people keep prescription drugs for several years (just in case they may need them again). When you borrow their meds, you have no way of knowing if you are taking a medication that has expired or has been stored under improper conditions.

➢ When your doctor is prescribing a certain medication for you, he is giving you a specific drug for a specific reason in a specific dose for a specific amount of time. He is aware of your drug allergies and any other bad reactions you may have had to medications in the past. Your doctor is also aware of the other medications you are taking, including prescription drugs, herbals, dietary supplements, and over-the-counter meds. Any of these other medications could interact with the new drug and cause serious harm.

➢ Self-medicating with someone else's drugs and bypassing the pharmacist's double-check is very risky and can lead to serious medication errors. When your pharmacist fills your prescription, he or she checks to make sure you are getting the right drug in the right dose at the right time. The pharmacist verifies that you know the name of the drug, what it is used for, how to take the medication, and what side effects to expect. The pharmacist will provide you with verbal instructions as well as written information to take home.

Bottom Line

Self-diagnosis and self-treatment with someone else's medications is risky and very dangerous. Don't do it. Call your doctor for help.

Safety Tip #55
I Can't Swallow My Pills:
When It's Not Safe to Crush
or Chew Your Tablets

Many people, especially those who have difficulty swallowing large tablets, find it convenient to crush tablets and mix them in applesauce or pudding. Sometimes crushing, chewing, or splitting tablets can lead to very serious and harmful effects. Always check with your pharmacist first.

Do Not Crush or Chew!

Stephanie was the caregiver for her dad who was suffering from lung cancer and was in a great deal of pain. To help him control it, the doctor gave him a new pain pill. The doctor told Stephanie the name of the new drug was Oxycontin used to treat chronic or long-term pain. The doctor told Stephanie it would slowly release the pain medicine into his body, so he was to take one pill every twelve hours. He also recommended she watch her dad for side effects including sleepiness, upset stomach, or constipation.

Stephanie knew what she would do. She would add the pain pill to her dad's meds in the morning and in the evening. Her dad had trouble swallowing, so to help him, Stephanie would crush them up and mix them in applesauce. This time, before Stephanie added the pain pills to her dad's regular meds, she read the label on the prescription bottle. The label stated, "Take one tablet by mouth every 12 hours for pain." There was a bright red sticker on the bottle that read "Do Not Crush or Chew."

Stephanie stopped and called the pharmacist for help. She asked the pharmacist if she could crush the Oxycontin and give it to her dad in applesauce with the rest of his pills.

The pharmacist told Stephanie that Oxycontin must never be crushed, cut, broken, chewed, or dissolved. Oxycontin was meant to be swallowed whole, as it was made specifically to release the medication slowly, continuously, around-the-clock. Crushing Oxycontin would release the entire drug all at once into her father's body. Since Oxycontin was an extremely potent pain med, this could cause him to have a severe (potentially fatal) overdose.

Stephanie was glad she had read the prescription label and called the pharmacist for help before she crushed her dad's new pain pill.

R_xpert Advice

Here are some specific guidelines on medications that should not be crushed, chewed, or split.

Controlled-Release

Do not crush, chew, split, cut, break, or dissolve any medications that are called "controlled-release." You should ask your pharmacist if any of your pills are controlled-release.

Controlled-released products are meant to enter your system slowly, generally over a twelve- to twenty-four-hour period. Crushing, chewing, breaking, or splitting the slow-release pills can instantly release the entire amount of drug into your body. Severe and even fatal overdoses have resulted from crushing long-acting medications. Contact your pharmacist and ask if it is safe before you crush your tablets, especially if it has any of the following letters or descriptions after the drug name.

CR   Controlled Release

ER   Extended Release

XR	Extended Release
XT	Extended Release
XL	Extended Release
LA	Long-Acting
CD	Controlled Delivery
SA	Sustained Action
SR	Sustained Release or Slow Release
Contin	Controlled Release
12 hour	Slow Release
24 hour	Slow Release

Following are some examples of controlled-release drugs:

Adderall XR

Augmentin XR

Cardene SR

Cardizem CD

Cardizem LA

Claritin-D 24 Hour

Special Coating

Some drugs have a special coating on them called *enteric coating* and are designated with the letters *EC*. Enteric coating protects you from stomach upset and helps the drug to be absorbed more effectively. These may include aspirin and other anti-inflammatory drugs. Check with your pharmacist before crushing drugs with an enteric coating.

Following are some examples of enteric-coated drugs:

Bayer EC

EC-Naprosyn

Entocort EC

Bottom Line

Ask your pharmacist if it is safe to crush, chew, split, break, cut, or dissolve any of your medications. This is especially true if you are taking controlled release or enteric-coated medications.

Safety Tip #56
Protect Your Pills: The Proper
Way to Store Medications

Many people store their medications in the bathroom "medicine cabinet," however, this is not the best location. Heat and moisture from shower or bathtub can cause pills to break down and lose their potency (strength). If a drug is starting to crumble, if the color is starting to change, or if it smells foul, do not take it. The medication has gone bad due to poor storage conditions. Taking medications that have gone bad could be harmful and endanger your health.

Her Headache Just Got Worse!

Linda had a headache. She needed to take some aspirin for the pain. She went to her bathroom medicine cabinet where she kept her medications. She opened the bottle and noticed a foul odor. She also noticed that some of the aspirin tablets were slightly yellowed and starting to crumble and fall apart.

Linda looked at the expiration date on the bottle. The aspirin were still within date; they were supposed to be good. Linda realized that storing them in the hot, humid bathroom where she liked to take long, steamy showers, had caused her pills to disintegrate and go bad. Linda's headache just got worse since now she had to go to the drugstore and buy more aspirin. One thing was for sure, she would no longer store the pills in the bathroom; she would keep them in a cool, dry, dark place, to prevent this from happening again.

R_xpert Advice

➢ Don't store your medications in the bathroom "medicine cabinet." The heat and humidity from the shower or tub can cause tablets to break down, crumble, and lose their potency. The heat and humidity can also cause capsules and gelcaps to become soft and stick together.

➢ If there are children in the house, store all medications (prescription and over-the-counter) in a locked drawer or cabinet.

➢ Keep all medications in their original container. The amber (yellow) color of the prescription bottle helps keep out light and can help prevent breakdown of the drug. If you take nitroglycerin for chest pain, keep the nitroglycerin tablets in the original glass, brown bottle with the tight screw cap it came in. The brown bottle and tight cap helps keep out light, air, and humidity. This helps prevent breakdown of the nitroglycerin tabs and is very important if you are having chest pains.

➢ Don't leave medications in your car or glove compartment where temperatures can rise well above the outside temperature or fall below a safe temperature and freeze. This will affect the potency of the drug.

➢ Don't take a medication that looks different than when you first took it. If a tablet has changed in size, shape, color, or smell, throw it away.

➢ If you need to refrigerate a medication, like insulin or children's liquid antibiotics, make sure they are stored where they will not get too warm or too cold and freeze. If you store medications in the refrigerator, be sure to keep them in an area where children will not be able to reach them.

➢ Never take a medication after it has expired. Some drugs may lose their strength, while other drugs actually start to break down. How a drug deteriorates after it expires is dependent on the drug itself and can change from one drug to another. Make it a practice to dispose of all drugs safely after they have expired.

➢ Storing your medications in a pillbox is great to help you stay organized; however, a regular pillbox is not airtight, light resistant, or childproof. Put enough medication in the pillbox for one week and keep the rest stored safely away.

➢ Don't store several different medications in one bottle. You may become confused as to which is which.

➢ If you think that one of your medications has gone bad, call your pharmacist. Do not take that medication without checking with your pharmacist first.

Bottom Line

Store all medications in a dry, dark, and cool, locked cabinet or drawer. Don't take a tablet or capsule that is starting to crumble, has changed shape or color, or smells foul.

Safety Tip #57
Health Hazard! Proper Disposal of Prescription Drugs

It used to be that as pharmacists, we always told people to dispose of any unused medications by pouring them down the drain or flushing them down the toilet. Now we know that this method, although effective in removing meds from the home, poses a threat to the environment.

It is important to get rid of any unused, unwanted, or expired medications as soon as possible. Removing these drugs from the home can prevent someone from taking them by accident, including small children and pets. It also discourages someone from finding them and selling them illegally.

Protect your loved ones and keep the environment safe by using the proper method for prescription drug disposal.

Got Drugs?

Sally had a job to do, and she was not looking forward to it. Several months ago her father had passed away, leaving behind a cabinet full of unused prescription medications. Sally did not know what to do with them. She knew not to flush them down the toilet or pour them down the drain, but how else was she supposed to get rid of it all?

Sally called her pharmacist for help. The pharmacist told her she was correct in not flushing the meds since they could get into the water supply and harm the environment. He also told her that she was right in wanting to get them out of the house, as they might become the target for theft.

The pharmacist told Sally about an upcoming drug "take-back" day called "Got Drugs?" that was sponsored by the FDA. He gave her the link to the FDA website so that she could find the date of the program and the nearest location.

Sally was able to drop off all of the old and unused prescription medications on the designated day at a location near her home. She was glad to be able to get rid of the drugs in a safe and environmentally friendly way.

Rxpert Advice

➢ Do not flush your medications down the toilet or pour them down the sink or drain. Most drugs can be thrown away safely in the trash after taking a few simple steps.

  1) Take the prescription drugs out of their original prescription bottle.

  2) Put the pills or capsules in a sealable plastic bag or a disposable container with a lid (such as an empty margarine tub).

  3) Mix the drugs with used coffee grounds, cat litter, or sawdust. This will make it less appealing to children and pets.

  4) Black out personal information on the prescription bottles with a black marker. This includes your name and prescription number.

  5) Put the sealed container or bags and the empty prescription bottles in the trash (do not put them into the recycle bin).

➢ Some pharmacies are starting to accept medications back from the pubic as a community service. Check with your pharmacy to see if they have a prescription drug take-back program.

> ➢ Find out if there is a special collection for unused and expired drugs in your community. Call your city or county government household trash and recycling service and ask if there is a drug take-back program available in your community.

> ➢ Got Drugs? is a national drug take-back program sponsored by the US Drug Enforcement Administration (DEA). This program happens several times a year. The DEA operates sites where you can drop off old or unneeded prescription drugs. There are more than four thousand drop-off locations nationwide, including many at local law enforcement offices. This service is free and completely anonymous—no questions asked. To find a collection site near you go to www.dea.gov, click on "Got Drugs?" and then following the links to enter your zip code.

> ➢ There are certain drugs that the Food and Drug Administration (FDA) does recommend you flush down the toilet or pour down the drain (see "Bonus" below to get a list of them). These drugs are especially harmful, even fatal, if they are taken by someone who is not meant to take them. Getting rid of these medications down the sink or drain is the best way to immediately and permanently remove the risk of accidental ingestion from your home.

Bottom Line

Protect your loved ones and the environment by taking a few simple steps to dispose of your unused, unwanted, or expired prescription medications safely.

Bonus

Go to www.drmarysue.com for a list of drugs the FDA wants you to flush.

Safety Tip #58
"Natural" Does Not
Always Mean "Safe"

Many people think that if the product says that it is "natural" that it must be "safe." This is not true. Don't be fooled into thinking that because a natural supplement or herbal product comes from a plant that it is safe for you to take. In fact, many of these natural supplements have serious side effects or could even interact with the prescription drugs you are taking.

Life-Threatening Effects

Stacey had been diagnosed with depression several years before and had been taking sertraline all along. This had always worked well for her, but lately she had been feeling down. Her friend told her she should try Saint-John's-wort, since she had taken it and it worked well for her depression.

Stacey went to the nutrition center and bought the Saint-John's-wort. She took it home and took the first dose that night along with her sertraline. Several days later, Stacey noticed that something was wrong. She felt anxious and jittery, her heart was fluttering in her chest, and she was shivering. What could be wrong?

Stacey called her doctor who told her to come in right away. The doctor asked Stacey what meds she was taking, and she told him about taking the Saint-John's-wort with the sertraline. She told him that she thought it would help her depression. The doctor was concerned, as he had seen cases before where Saint-John's-wort interacted with other drugs for depression, causing similar symptoms to what Stacey was experiencing.

The doctor told Stacey to stop taking the Saint-John's-wort. He told her the jitteriness, shivering, and heart problems should go away within the next few days. Stacey knew now never to start taking herbal remedies without talking to her doctor or pharmacist first—there were too many serious problems that could happen.

R_xpert Advice

Prescription drugs and over-the-counter meds are tested and proven safe and effective before reaching the market. Herbal products and natural supplements do not undergo the same testing and are not proven either safe or effective before you take them.

➢ Herbal products and natural supplements may not be pure. They may contain products that are not on the label and may be harmful for you.

➢ Herbal products and natural supplements are advertised to treat a variety of different ailments; however, there is very little evidence to support claims that these supplements actually work. Anecdotes and testimonials are often the only information available for consumers.

➢ Do not take herbal products or natural supplements if you are elderly, have blood-clotting problems, cancer, diabetes, enlarged prostate, epilepsy, glaucoma, heart disease, high blood pressure, immune system problems, psychiatric problems, Parkinson's disease, liver problems, stroke or thyroid problems.

➢ If you are scheduled for surgery, stop taking herbal products or natural supplements two weeks prior to your procedure. Some of these may cause bleeding or problems with anesthesia.

➢ Always tell your doctor if you are taking any natural products or supplements.

➢ Side effects of herbal products and natural supplements range from upset stomach and dry mouth to headache, feeling nervous, and an uneven heartbeat. If you think you are having a side effect to a natural product, check with your doctor or pharmacist.

> ➤ Herbal products and natural supplements interfere with many prescription drugs. Do not use herbal products or natural supplements if you are also taking drugs for depression, seizures, blood thinners, high blood pressure, HIV/AIDS, heart disease, diabetes, or cancer. Herbal products or natural supplements may decrease the effectiveness of your prescription medication.

> ➤ Do not take more that the recommended dose of a natural product or herbal supplement.

> ➤ Do not take a natural product or herbal supplement if you are pregnant or nursing.

> ➤ Only take natural products or herbal supplements under the guidance of a trained medical professional.

Bottom Line

Don't assume that because a supplement says "natural" that it is safe. Check with your doctor or pharmacist before taking any natural product or herbal supplement.

Bonus

Go to www.drmarysue.com for a list of prescription and herbal drug interactions.

Safety Tip #59
"New, Revolutionary, Super-Enhanced, Extreme" Dietary Supplements

If it sounds too good to be true, it is. In fact, the "new, revolutionary, ultimate, extreme, super-enhanced" dietary supplement you saw advertised on TV, the radio, the Internet, e-mail, or at the local health food store, could be very dangerous.

"Dietary supplements" encompass those products sold for weight-loss, sexual enhancement, bodybuilding, prostate "health," youthfulness, mood enhancement, and other reasons. Because these products are considered *food* supplements and not *drugs*, the government allows manufacturers to market supplements without proving that they are either safe or effective. As long as supplements do not claim to treat, prevent, or cure a specific disease, they can enter and stay on the market. Remember, if it sounds too good to be true, it is. Don't fall for exaggerated and unfounded claims. Save your money and your health.

Wow! That Sounds Too Good to Be True!

James was getting on in years. Every time he saw his doctor, he gave him another prescription. He never felt any different and he was tired of taking all of those prescription drugs. His friend told him about some dietary supplements that would help him regain some of that youthful feeling. He decided to go to the health food store to check these out. He asked the girl at the counter for help.

James told the clerk that he had high blood pressure and his prescription medications didn't seem to make any difference. The clerk told him to stop taking the prescription drugs and start taking garlic instead. It would help his blood pressure and it was totally safe. That sounded too good to be true! James would get a bottle.

Then James told her that he was having memory problems and that the doctor had prescribed a pill for it. The clerk told him that he could stop taking that and take ginkgo biloba. It really helped your memory. James got some of that too!

Wow, thought James, *these supplements can really help me.* He bought several other products on the way out.

Three days later, James was admitted to the hospital. He had passed out when his blood pressure had gotten out of control. James's doctor was confused and very concerned since James was well controlled on his medications and had never had any problems before. James admitted to the doctor that he had stopped taking his prescription blood pressure medication and had started taking garlic. He also told him that he had stopped the memory drug and tried gingko instead.

The doctor was not happy with James. He told him to start taking his prescription drugs as he was supposed to and stop the supplements. They were obviously not working and had been the cause of his admission to the hospital. He told him in the future to stay away from all supplements and to let him do his job and prescribe safe and effective medications for him. James would do exactly that. He had learned the hard way that if it sounds too good to be true, it is.

R_xpert Advice

- ➢ Never take a dietary supplement without talking to your doctor or pharmacist first. They will tell you whether it is safe and effective.

- ➢ Do not take supplements that claim to act like and be as effective as the prescription drug. Claims like this are impossible to validate.

- ➢ Do not take supplements with labeling in a foreign language.

➢ Do not take supplements marketed through mass e-mails, the Internet, or on the radio.

➢ Do not seek medical advice from untrained store clerks. It is their job to sell you these supplements whether they work or not. If you buy these supplements, you will be out a lot of money for an ineffective product that potentially could cause you harm.

➢ Do not take supplements that claim to be legal versions of bodybuilding steroids. It is nearly impossible to identify what (if any) drug is in these products.

➢ Do not take supplements that promise fast sexual effects that last for hours. This is unproven and could be dangerous.

Bottom Line

Before you buy and take a dietary supplement, ask your doctor or pharmacist if it is safe for you to take and if it is really effective. Most of the time, the answer will be no. Save your money.

Safety Tip #60
The Unsung Hero: The Caregiver at Home

Caring for a loved one at home is a demanding and challenging situation. Providing the necessary care for daily activities from bathing and toileting, to meal preparation and general care is hard enough, but giving the correct medications at the right time in the right doses can be confusing and overwhelming.

Greased Lightning

My mother was the caregiver and advocate for my stepfather for more than ten years. He suffered from Parkinson's disease, including dementia, and was homebound for the last ten years of his life. One day, my mom asked me to watch my stepdad for a few hours while she ran a few errands. I agreed and showed up at the designated time. Mom had just given my stepdad his morning meds, and she told me that he would not need any more until she returned.

My stepdad and I settled in to watch an afternoon of C-SPAN, which always held his attention; however, it put me right to sleep. I kept forcing myself to stay awake, but ultimately the drone from the TV and the eighty-degree temperature in their house knocked me out.

I was only asleep for a few minutes (I promise) when I heard a noise coming from the kitchen. To my surprise, my stepdad had gotten out of his chair and was quickly moving about the kitchen. This was the fastest I'd seen him move in months. He was like greased lightning!

Then I saw what he was doing. He had his pillbox in his hand and several of the compartments were open. There were pills scattered on the counter and some on the floor. It was clear to me that he had taken some of the pills.

At that exact moment, the back door opened, and my mom came in the house. "What is going on?" she asked me. "I thought you were going to watch him."

"I just shut my eyes for a few minutes, and he moved so quickly and quietly he took me totally by surprise." I had no idea that my stepdad could get into so much trouble so fast!

My mom was mad, but she agreed that once my stepdad got something in his head there was no stopping him. He had patiently waited for me to shut my eyes and then he moved into action. Now I knew better—I'd never be fooled again. The next time Mom asked me to watch him, I'd be sure to put something on TV besides C-SPAN and keep my eyes on him at all times.

R$_x$pert Advice

> ➢ In the role of the caregiver, giving medications is serious business. Above all, it takes preparation and organization. Remember NUTS and talk to the pharmacist about any concerns you have regarding your loved one's medications.

> ➢ Your pharmacist can review the medication list and tell you if there are any drugs that should not be given together and help you create an easier dosing schedule. A clear, efficient medication schedule will help you to give the meds on time and in the right order. Place a check mark next to each med after giving it, so if you become distracted, you will be able to see whether you have given a med or not.

> ➢ Ask your pharmacist about using a pillbox or other reminder system to keep track of the medications. Fill it once a week. Keep it locked and store it out of sight and out of reach, so your "patient" can't get to it.

➤ Keep track of your loved one's medical records by using the Personal Health System (PHS). Make it easy on yourself by asking the receptionist at the doctor's office to punch holes in the reports and instructions your doctor gives you, and then you can insert them in the PHS binder before you leave the office. Do the same thing when you receive reports in the mail: simply use a three-hole punch and put them in the PHS under the designated tab.

Bottom Line

As the caregiver, in addition to everything else that you do, it is up to you to find a way to give medications as safely and accurately as possible. Ask your doctor and pharmacist for help if you do not understand how to give a medication so that you can prevent a serious medication error from happening to your loved one. Keep medicines out of sight and out of reach of a loved one in your care.

Epilogue: Patient-Centered Care

A new model of health care is emerging in our hospitals and outpatient health-care settings called "Patient Centered Care." It means that the patient is the center of his or her health-care team. Patients and their caregivers or advocates are actively involved in decisions about their own care. These decisions encompass the total needs of the patient rather than just focusing on the disease or illness itself. It is expected that patients will take an active role and responsibility for the coordination of their own health care by keeping up-to-date records and communicating concerns with their doctors, nurses, pharmacists, and other providers.

"We're In This Together"

Recently, I was asked to appear on a local TV news program to talk about medication errors. The reporter presented statistics about the high rate of medication errors and asked what consumers could do to prevent them from happening. I talked about the need for health-care consumers to take an active role in their care by asking the four simple questions and remembering NUTS. I talked about look-alike and sound-alike medications and how easy it was for doctors and nurses to become confused by similar sounding drug names. I talked about the need for consumers with common last names to stop and make sure that they received the right drugs before leaving the pharmacy. I asked that the consumer open their prescription bag before leaving the prescription counter to make sure they received the correct medications.

The next day, several colleagues at the hospital where I work remarked about the TV news program and about how I was getting the word out about medication safety. "We're in this together," said one of the patient-safety nurses. "People need to know that we need them to take an active role in their own care. We rely on them to tell us important information about their illnesses. They need to work with us to be certain that we have all of the information we need and that they are getting the right medications and the safest care possible." These colleagues encouraged me to continue getting the word out and to continue to motivate people to take a central role in their own health care.

Preventing Medication Errors in a "NUTShell"

- ➤ If it doesn't seem right, it probably isn't.
- ➤ Never assume anything.
- ➤ Ask the four NUTS questions—and get the answers you need and can understand.
- ➤ Keep an updated medication list.
- ➤ Stay organized and keep a Personal Health System.

Bottom Line

By taking the steps outlined in this book, partnering with your doctor, pharmacist, and other health-care providers, learning to ask questions, and keeping all of your records current and in one place, you are taking a very big step in preventing medication errors and ensuring the highest quality and safety of your health care.

Bonus

Bookmark my website to stay up to date and get resources you need today: www.drmarysue.com. You will find the Personal Health Care System binder as well as forms you can download and up-to-date information about different diseases, illnesses, and new drugs.

Reliable Medical Resources

You or someone you care for has just been given a new medication. Take some time to read about that new medication, and if you have any questions, ask your doctor or pharmacist for help. The following websites and resources are provided for educational purposes only and are not to be used in place of medical advice, diagnosis, treatment recommendations, or referrals to practitioners.

For Drug Information

MedlinePlus: A service of the US National Library of Medicine and the National Institutes of Health that provides information on prescription and over-the-counter medications—http://www.nlm.nih.gov/medlineplus/druginformation.html
US Food and Drug Administration Center for Drug Evaluation and Research: Provides information on prescription and over-the-counter medications, consumer drug information, reports, and publications—http://www.fda.gov/cder. Main FDA for general inquiries: 1-888-INFO-FDA (1-888-463-6332). Drug Information: 1-301-827-4570. To submit a report about Adverse Drug Reaction: Medwatch: 1-800-FDA-1088.

Drugs.com: Provides information on nearly twenty-four thousand different prescription drugs, over-the-counter meds, and natural products, including pill identification, drug interaction checker, and side effects http://www.drugs.com.

United States Pharmacopeia (USP): an official public standards-setting authority for all prescription and over-the-counter medicines and other health-care products—http://www.usp.org.

NCCAM Clearinghouse: provides information on complementary and alternative medicine—http://www.nccam.nih.gov. Toll-free in the United States: 1-888-644-6226. TTY (for deaf and hard-of-hearing callers): 1-866-464-3615. E-mail: info@nccam.nih.gov.

PubMed: A service of the National Library of Medicine (NLM), it provides summaries of articles from scientific and medical journals—http://www.ncbi.nlm.nih.gov/entrez.

Cochrane Database: The information on this website summarizes the results of clinical trials on health-care treatments. (Summaries are free. Full-text articles require a subscription.)—http://www.cochrane.org.

VIPPS (Verified Internet Pharmacy Practice Sites): The VIPPS symbol signifies public accountability of the pharmacy and the commitment to the patient's health and safety. Check out this website before ordering medications online—http://www.nabp.net/programs/accreditation/vipps/.

Quality Check: The Joint Commission on the Accreditation of Healthcare Organization's search engine to locate accredited health-care organizations in the United States. Visitors can search by city and state, by name, or by zip code http://www.qualitycheck.org/consumer/searchQCR.aspx.

Hospital Compare: This website allows patients to compare and find the best hospitals in the United States based on several indicators—http://www.hospitalcompare.hhs.gov.

Healthgrades: A private organization designed to provide ratings and profiles of hospitals, nursing homes, and physicians—http://www.healthgrades.com.

Consumers Advancing Patient Safety (CAPS): Promotes a partnership between you and your doctors—http://www.patientsafety.org/.

Drug-Discount Card Programs

Many pharmaceutical companies offer discount cards that can save you money each year. Check out these sites to find out which one is the best one for you.

✓ Johnson and Johnson Partnership for Prescription Assistance—http://www.pparx.org. Phone: 1-888-4PPA-NOW

- ✓ Pfizer Pfriends Program—http://www.pfizerhelpfulanswers. com. Phone: 1-866-776-3700
- ✓ U Share Prescription Drug Discount Card—http://www. usharerx.com. Phone: 1-800-707-3917
- ✓ AstraZeneca Foundation Patient-Assistance Program— http://www.astrazeneca-us.com. Phone: 1-800-424-3727
- ✓ Lilly Answers—http://www.lillyanswers.com/en/index. html. Phone: 1-877-RX-LILLY
- ✓ Janssen Patient Assistance Program—http://www. janssen.com. Phone: 1-800-652-6227
- ✓ Medicare-Approved Drug Discount Cards—http:// www.medicare.gov. Phone: 1-800-MEDICARE
- ✓ Together Rx Access—http://www.trxaccess.com. Phone: 1-800-444-4106

Medication Safety Websites

These websites focus on educating the consumer and the healthcare provider about medication errors and patient safety.

- ✓ Institute for Safe Medication Practices—http://www. ismp.org
- ✓ The Joint Commission on the Accreditation of Healthcare Organizations—http://www.jointcommission.org
- ✓ Agency for Healthcare Research and Quality—Medical Error and Patient Safety—http://www.ahrq.gov
- ✓ American Society of Health-System Pharmacists— Patient Safety Resource Center—http://www.ashp.org/ patientsafety
- ✓ Citizens for Patient Safety—http:// citizensforpatientsafety.org/
- ✓ Institute for Healthcare Improvement—http://www.ihi.org
- ✓ Institute of Medicine—http://www.iom.edu
- ✓ National Patient Safety Foundation—http://www.npsf.org

- ✓ National Coordinating Council on Medication Error Reporting and Prevention—http://www.nccmerp.org
- ✓ National Council on Patient Information and Education—http://talkaboutrx.org/
- ✓ National Quality Forum—http://www.qualityforum.org/Home.aspx
- ✓ Patient Safety and Quality Healthcare—http://www.psqh.com
- ✓ Partnership for Patient Safety—http://p4ps.net/Home.html/
- ✓ Safety Leaders—http://www.safetyleaders.org

Medication List

Name: _____

Date:_____

Medication Allergies or Reactions: _____

_____

Name of Pharmacy: _____

Phone Number of Pharmacy:_____

Start Date	Name of medicine*	Use	How I Take This Medication	Side Effects	Stop Date

*Include all vitamins, herbal supplements, nutritional products, antacids, laxatives, allergy relief products, and other over-the-counter medications.

Emergency Health Profile........<inline>Page 1 of 4</inline>

Full Name:_____

Address: _____

City: _____ State:_____

Zip:_____

Home Phone:_____

Cell Phone: _____

Date of birth: _____ Age: _____

Social Security Number:_____

Primary Language Spoken: _____

Sex: ☐   Male ☐   Female

Race:_____ Weight:_____ Height: _____

Blood Type:_____

List all of your Medical Problems:

_____

_____

<u>List all allergies to medications and food</u>:

_____

_____

<u>Who to Call in an Emergency</u>:

1) Name:_____

Relationship to you: _____

Home Phone number: _____

Cell Phone number: _____

Work Phone number: _____

<u>Doctor's Information</u>:

Primary Care Doctor's Name: _____

Primary Care Doctor's Phone Number:_____

<u>List all of the medications you are taking. Be sure to include all</u>
<u>over-the-counter drugs</u>.

Name of your drugstore: _____

Phone number of drugstore: _____

Start Date	Name of medicine*	Use	How I Take This Medication	Side Effects	Stop Date

List all of your medical appliances (hearing aid, dentures, pacemaker, insulin pump, glasses, contact lenses etc.): _____

_____

<u>Insurance Information:</u>

Name of Health Insurance: _____

Name of Policy holder: _____

Plan: _____

Insurance company customer service phone number: _____

Member ID: _____

Policy number: _____

Group: _____

Other insurance information:_____

Important Information that you would want the Emergency Room Doctor to Know:_____

Date form prepared:_____

Prepared by:_____

Acknowledgments

I would like to acknowledge the "leading role" that Dennis and Kimberly Quaid have played in bringing the issue of medication errors to the public spotlight following the near-fatal heparin overdose of their newborn twins in 2007. Their children survived that error and Dennis Quaid, in partnership with Dr. Charles Denham, TMIT, and Safetyleaders.org, has gone on to be an advocate and international spokesperson for safer medication practices. That medication error made me say, "Enough is enough" and motivated me to write this book.

I also would like to thank the many people who shared their medication error stories with me and allowed me to use them in this book. Their stories will go on to help others by illustrating how easily these mistakes can happen to just about anyone.

Special thanks go to Robin Hoffman, GetPublishedCoach. com for her unique brand of encouragement and in teaching me the importance of a story in explaining difficult and complicated medical information to everyday health-care consumers.

Lastly, I would like to thank my husband, Keith, for never failing to dispense large doses of expert advice "prn" and to my children, Chip, John, and especially Katie, for their encouragement and support.

Notes

1. IOM (Institute of Medicine), "To Err Is Human: Building a Safer Health System" (Washington DC: National Academy Press, 1999).

2. Lucian L. Leape and Donald M. Berwick, "Five Years after To Err Is Human: What Have We Learned?" *JAMA* 293, no. 19 (May 18, 2005).

3. "To Err Is Human—To Delay Is Deadly. Ten Years Later, a Million Lives Lost, Billions of Dollars Wasted." http://www.safepatientproject.org/safepatientproject.org/pdf/safepatientproject.org-ToDelayIsDeadly.pdf (accessed May 3, 2009).

4. IOM, "To Err Is Human," 1999.

5. IOM (Institute of Medicine), "Preventing Medication Errors" (Washington DC: National Academy Press, 2007).

6. IOM, "To Err Is Human," 1999.

7. Ibid.

8. Joint Commission on the Accreditation of Healthcare Organizations—Speak Up Program. http://www.jointcommission.org/speakup.aspx (accessed January 10, 2010).

9. Michael Roizen and Mehmet Oz, *YOU: The Smart Patient: An Insider's Handbook for Getting the Best Treatment* (New York: Free Press, 2006).

10. Consumer Reports Health Poll, "Two-Thirds of Americans Say Drug Makers Have Too Much Sway over Doctors; Information about Safety and Side Effects Sorely Needed." http://www.prnewswire. com/news-releases/consumer-reports-health (accessed September 12, 2010).

11. J. Donohue, M. Cevasco, and M. Rosenthal, "A Decade of Direct-to-Consumer Advertising of Prescription Drugs," *New England Journal of Medicine* 357 (August 16, 2007): 673–681. Accessed October 4, 2009.

12. "ISMP Medication Safety Alert—Treat Medication Samples with Respect." http://www.ismp.org/ Newsletters/consumer/alerts/Samples.asp (accessed December 14, 2010).

13. Committee on Identifying and Preventing Medication Errors, Institute of Medicine, IOM (Institute of Medicine), "Preventing Medication Errors" (Washington DC: National Academy Press, 2007).

14. Davis, et al.,"Literacy and Misunderstanding Prescription Drug Labels," *Annals of Internal Medicine* (November 2006).

15. "Double Trouble—Consumer Awareness of Look-alike Names Is Critical for Drug Safety," (September/ October 2010). http://www.consumermedsafety.org.

16. Tim Fagan's Law H.R. 4076. http://www. opencongress.org/bill/110-h4076/show.

17. IOM, "Preventing Medication Errors," 2007.

18. IOM, "To Err Is Human," 1999.

19. Roizen and Oz, *YOU: The Smart Patient.*

20. "The Granny Syndrome," ConsumerMedSafety.org.

21. "Keep out of reach of children." http://www.tylenol.com.

22. "Generation Rx: National Study Confirms Abuse of Prescription and Over-the-Counter Drugs," Partnership for a Drug-Free America (May 15, 2006). http://www.drugfree.org/portal/drugissue/research/teens_2005/Generation_Rx_Study_Confirms_Abuse_of_Prescription (accessed November 7, 2010).

23. "Fact Sheet: Prescription Drug Abuse—A DEA Focus." http://www.usdoj.gov/dea/good_medicine_bad_behavior_factsheet.doc. (accessed November 7, 2010).

www.ingramcontent.com/pod-product-compliance
Lightning Source LLC
Chambersburg PA
CBHW031836170526
45157CB00001B/316